The Management of Head Injuries

Second edition

David G. Currie
Consultant Neurosurgeon
Aberdeen Royal Infirmary

with

Ewan Ritchie
Consultant Anaesthetist
Perth Royal Infirmary

Stephen Stott
Consultant Anaesthetist
Aberdeen Royal Infirmary

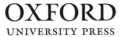

OXFORD
UNIVERSITY PRESS

OXFORD

UNIVERSITY PRESS

Great Clarendon Street, Oxford OX2 6DP

Oxford   New York

Athens Auckland Bangkok Bogota Bombay Buenos Aires
Calcutta Cape Town Dar es Salaam Delhi Florence Hong Kong Istanbul
Karachi Kuala Lumpur Madras Madrid Melbourne Mexico City
Nairobi Paris São Paulo Singapore Taipei Tokyo Toronto Warsaw

and associated companies in

Berlin Ibadan

Oxford is a trade mark of Oxford University Press

First Edition published 1993
Second Edition published 2000

A catalogue record for this title is available from the British Library
Library of Congress Cataloging in Publication Data
Currie, David G.
The management of head injuries/David G. Currie, Ewan Ritchie,
Stephen Stott, – 2nd ed.
Includes bibliographical references and index.
1. Head – Wounds and injuries Handbooks, manuals, etc.
I. Ritchie, Ewan, II. Stott, Stephen. III. Title.
[DNLM: 1. Brain Injuries – therapy Handbooks. 2. Head Injuries –
therapy Handbooks. WL 39 C976m 2000]
RD521.C86 2000   617.5′1044–dc21   99–36446

1 3 5 7 9 10 8 6 4 2

ISBN 0 19 263078 4

Typeset by EXPO Holdings, Malaysia

Printed by Thomson Press, India

Preface to the first edition

Head injury is a common problem, and one which is dealt with very largely by non-specialists, often by junior doctors and often in district hospitals where specialist neurosurgical assistance is lacking. This book is intended to be a guide for the junior doctor working in the Accident and Emergency Department or the Orthopaedic or General Surgical Ward. The emphasis is on the early management of the head-injured patient. The chapter on 'Operative surgery' has been written in the knowledge that the isolated general surgeon may, on occasions, be required to operate on head-injured patients when transfer to a specialist centre is impossible.

This is very much a practical handbook, and not a substitute for the excellent textbooks on the subject which are currently available and are referred to in Further reading.

Aberdeen   D. G. C.
February 1993

Preface to the second edition

The first edition of this book was introduced as a handbook for doctors and nurses in the 'frontline' providing early treatment for head-injured patients. This remains the purpose of the second edition. Only a minority of head-injured patients are cared for by neurosurgeons. The majority of the very large number of head-injured patients seen in hospitals each year are cared for initially by junior doctors in Accident and Emergency and other surgical specialties. The crucial task of recognizing neurological deterioration in the head-injured is undertaken by nurses in various surgical specialties. Chapter 11 on managing the disturbed head-injured patient was included at the suggestion of nursing colleagues who have to bear the brunt of this difficult task.

Anaesthetists also play a major part in the care of the resuscitation, transportation, and intensive care of head-injured patients and two anaesthetists have contributed to this edition by revising the chapters on transport (Chapter 13) and resuscitation (Chapter 3), and by addition of a chapter on anaesthesia in head injuries (Chapter 10), Chapter 7 on cervical spine injuries has been expanded. The essential message remains the same—good resuscitation, skilled observation, and timely action in the event of deterioration by those who look after head-injured patients in the early stages provide the best chance of a favourable outcome.

Aberdeen and Perth
D. G. C.
E. R.
S. S.

Publishers Note
The publishers would like to thank Dr Colin Robertson for his valuable advice during the preparation of this book.

Contents

1 Introduction

Epidemiology

In Scotland, with a population of approximately 5 million people, 80 000 to 90 000 patients are seen each year following injuries to the head. This gives an attendance rate of 1600 to 1800 per 100 000 of the population. The attendance rate in the United States is almost double this figure. Head-injured patients are seen initially by junior doctors in Accident and Emergency (A&E) departments in district general hospitals and teaching hospitals, and by general practitioners in community hospitals. On the basis of this initial assessment approximately 20 000 patients are admitted to hospital annually in Scotland. A similar proportion, 300 to 400 per 100 000 of the population, is admitted to hospital in England and Wales. The patterns of aetiology, attendance rate, and admission rate vary in other European countries, as does the influence of alcohol. There is a wide variation in the nature of the admitting unit, which may be in a small isolated district hospital on the one hand, or in a major teaching hospital on the other.

The care of head-injured patients is by general surgeons, orthopaedic surgeons, and A&E specialists in most instances. Only a miniority are admitted directly to neurosurgical wards. In Scotland, less than 1000 patients are eventually admitted to neurosurgical units annually, and only a minority of this group require operative intervention by a neurosurgeon. This means that only 1% of all head-injured patients seen in the A&E department are admitted to neurosurgical units.

It is clear from these figures that a great deal of the decision making in the management of head injuries is done by non-specialists, and often by junior doctors in a variety of specialties. Given the ratio of neurosurgeons and neurosurgical beds to population in Britain, head-injured patients will continue to be cared for in this fashion, and the quality of service provided depends crucially on the education of non-specialists in the early assessment and subsequent management of the head-injured patient. The main possibilities for improvement in our management of head injuries lie not in the are of operative neurosurgery but in the organization of the early management of the patient in the A&E department, in the admitting ward, and in transit between the admitting unit and the specialist centre.

The doctor with primary responsibility for head injuries is faced with a series of decisions (Box 1.1).

The doctor on the spot is also faced with certain practical tasks, and may not always have the benefit of specialist advice immediately to hand. The assessment and resuscitation of the head-injured patient are the task of the receiving doctor in the A&E department, and cannot be deferred until specialist help is available. The interpretation of skull

Box 1.1   Decisions facing the doctor with primary responsibility for head injuries

- Who should have a skull X-ray?
- Who should be admitted to hospital?
- Who is at risk of an intracranial haematoma?
- Who should have a CT scan?
- Who should be transferred to a specialist centre?
- Who should be operated on at the base hospital?
- Who should be ventilated?

X-rays and the management of scalp injuries also fall to the doctor on the spot, and in some circumstances the skull injury and even the intracranial haematoma may need to be dealt with by the non-specialist.

Causes of head injury

Head injuries are twice as common in men as in women. The great majority of head injuries are caused by road traffic accidents, falls, and assaults (Box 1.2); but the proportion of injuries due to each cause varies according to age group. Falls and domestic accidents are much more common in the elderly, whereas assaults and industrial injuries are more common among younger men. Alcohol is the single commonest causative factor in head injury.

The aetiology of the accident is important in drawing attention to the possibility of associated injuries, and may be of medico-legal significance in an era of increasing litigation. It is essential to ask how the patient came to fall and strike the head. Where no obvious explanation is forthcoming it is possible that the accident was preceded by loss

Box 1.2   Causes of head injury

- Road-traffic accidents
- Falls
- Domestic accidents
- Recreational accidents
- Industrial accidents
- Assault
- Fits and other causes of loss of consciousness

of consciousness, and this will require investigation in its own right. The fall may have been the result of a fit, a cardiac arrhythmia, or an intracranial haemorrhage. The account of an eyewitness is important in establishing how the accident happened; and when an immediate eyewitness is not available the observations of the police or other emergency personnel may be helpful. Occasionally, for instance, a driver may be involved in a road traffic accident because of prior loss of consciousness. The police observations at the scene of the accident may raise this possibility. As well as supplying an explanation for the injury, the police, the ambulance crew, or other witnesses may be able to give valuable information about the patient's state of consciousness after the injury.

The nature of the head injury may also draw attention to the possible complications. The drunken patient, for instance, who falls forward and presents with a bleeding nose and black eyes is a prime candidate for an anterior cranial fossa fracture and cerebrospinal fluid (CSF) rhinorrhoea. The same injury may be complicated by a hyperextension injury of the neck and spinal cord trauma. A study of head-injured patients with altered consciousness at the time of admission to a neurosurgical unit has compared those injuries caused by high-velocity impacts (as in road traffic accidents) with those caused by low-velocity impacts (as in falls). In the case of high-velocity injuries there was a high incidence of multiple injuries, and, hence, a high incidence of extracranial complications, but only a 26% incidence of intracranial haematoma. In the case of low-velocity injury the incidence of extracranial complications was much lower, but the incidence of intracranial haematoma was 59%.

Penetrating head injuries are seen more frequently in warfare or in civil violence but they also occur sporadically as a result of assault, industrial injuries, and falls on to sharp objects. Once again, a careful history of the circumstances of the injury may draw attention to the possibility of a penetrating injury when the scalp injury appears innocuous. The consequences of penetrating injuries are serious but avoidable if recognized.

Head injury accounts for 26% of all deaths due to injury in the United States and 2% of all deaths. Head injuries account for only 1% of all deaths in Britain. Some 57% of all deaths from head injury in the United States are due to road traffic accidents, and 12% to falls. There is a bimodal distribution of deaths from head injury according to age group, with the peaks occurring in the age range 15–24 on the one hand, and in the age range over 75 years on the other.

Road traffic accidents

These accidents remain the commonest cause of severe head injury, and often form a component of multiple injuries in the same patient. The associated injuries commonly result in respiratory impairment or hypovolaemia, which, in turn, exacerbate the brain injury. Furthermore, the effects of respiratory impairment and hypovolaemia may be prolonged if the patient is trapped in the vehicle. In these circumstances it may be that a substantial proportion of the brain injury is due to systemic factors causing cerebral ischaemia and hypoxia, and only a relatively small part to the head injury itself.

Legislation to make the use of seat belts compulsory was introduced in Australia in 1970, with a dramatic reduction in both the death rate from road traffic accidents and the incidence of head injury. Seat belt legislation was introduced in Britain in 1983. One year later the death rate from road traffic accidents had fallen by 25%, and this was largely due to the prevention of severe head injuries. One study in Nottingham compared the incidence of injuries in the three months before legislation with that in the subsequent three months. There was a fall in the incidence of head injury of more than 50%, and a similar fall in the incidence of facial injuries. Compulsory seat belt legislation has been repealed in certain states in the United States, and in each case there has been a marked increase in the incidence of head injury.

Not only has the death rate fallen after seat belt legislation, but there has been a change in the pattern of head injury resulting from road traffic accidents. Before the wide-spread wearing of seat belts the unrestrained driver or passenger was thrown forwards, striking the windscreen with the head. This resulted in complex injuries of the head and face, together with scalp and facial lacerations. Compound, comminuted, and often depressed frontal fractures were seen, and the brunt of the brain injury was received by the frontal lobes. Some of the energy of the impact was absorbed as the frontal bones were fractured, thereby diminishing the force applied to the brain. Such a patient might require exploration and elevation of the frontal fractures, debridement of the damaged brain, maxillo-facial surgery, and possibly a tracheostomy. The survivors were left with disfiguring facial scars and intellectual impairment. Some suffered visual loss due to optic nerve injuries. The seat belted vehicle occupant involved in a similar accident is spared the complex, disfiguring frontal and facial injuries; but the brain injury may, paradoxically, be more severe. As the head is brought abruptly to rest, the energy derived from the loss of momentum is transmitted to the brain, causing diffuse damage rather than the localized damage described above.

Motor cycles and pedal cycles

Approximately 5000 serious injuries amongst pedal cyclists occur each year in Britain, with a 75% incidence of head injury. As a result, there are approximately 300 deaths each year. Pedal cyclists are more likely to suffer head injuries than those involved in motor cycle accidents, and those suffering from head injuries have a higher incidence of severe head injuries than motor cyclists. Experience in the United States, Germany, and Australia has shown that the use of cycling helmets brings about a very substantial reduction in serious head injury. The potential reduction in head injuries as a result of the use of cycling helmets has been estimated in different studies as being between 80 and 90%. Cycling accidents occur most frequently on main roads, and particularly at road junctions. Provision of cycle lanes or cycle tracks reduces the incidence of head injury.

Sports injuries

Head injury occurs in most sports. There is some discernible pattern from sport to sport. In contact sports, such as football and rugby, blunt head injury is caused by clashes of heads or kicks. Scalp and skull injuries are uncommon. Head injury is the commonest cause of death in climbing accidents; and since the head injury is so often fatal the numbers of head-injured climbers seen in hospital are surprisingly small, even in popular climbing areas. As in the case of road traffic accidents, injuries in climbing accidents are often multiple. Horse riding is the single most dangerous sport in the context of head injury. Some 33% of equestrian accidents include head injuries, and in 1983 there were 12 deaths in Britain. Studies of equestrian head injuries have shown a significant reduction in serious head injuries when protective headgear is worn. A British Standard for riding hats has been established.

Sports injuries account for 20–30% of children's head injuries. Surprisingly, the sport most frequently implicated in Britain is golf! The majority of children thus injured are struck as their friends swing the club. Skull fractures occur in the majority of these children, and in most cases these are depressed fractures requiring elevation.

Alcohol and head injury

Alcohol is an important factor both in the aetiology of head injury and as a complicating factor. It is particularly implicated in head injuries caused by falls and assaults, and in pedestrians injured in road traffic accidents; but irrespective of the cause of injury, alcohol intoxication is associated with a higher incidence of head injury than that found in sober victims of injury. In Finland, 64% of intoxicated patients presenting in A&E departments have head injuries, compared with 17% of sober accident victims.

In Scotland, 40–50% of patients admitted to hospital after head injury had recently taken alcohol.

The intoxicated patient is more likely to vomit and aspirate gastric contents. It is difficult to assess the extent to which the patient's conscious level is due to the head injury and how much to ascribe to alcohol. It is not uncommon for the relatives of head-injured patients to attribute the victim's drowsiness or failure to wake the next morning to his/her overindulgence on the previous night—indeed, it is not unknown in Scotland for the patient to be left 'to sleep it off' for more than 24 hours before it is realized that there is more to the stupor than can be ascribed to a hangover.

Since alcohol consumption is so common among head-injury victims impaired consciousness should never be attributed to the effects of alcohol alone. There is a poor correlation between conscious state and blood or breath alcohol levels, but experience in Glasgow has been that consciousness is not impaired until blood alcohol levels exceed 2 g/litre.

Pathophysiology of head injury

It is necessary to be aware of some theoretical concepts in order to appreciate the requirements of the head-injured patient.

Primary and secondary brain injury

The **primary brain injury** is that which is inflicted at the time of impact. It ranges from the minor concussional injury with brief loss of consciousness to the severe brain injury with prolonged coma or severe focal damage. The damage is established at the time of the impact, and is not amenable to surgical treatment. Recovery takes place, partially or completely depending on the severity of the brain injury, provided that a suitable environment is created to enable healing to proceed unhindered.

The **secondary brain injury** may follow at any time after the impact, and is due to a variety of potentially preventable or reversible causes such as intracranial haemorrhage, impaired respiration leading to hypoxia and hypercapnia, and decreased cerebral perfusion due to hypotension. The essence of head-injury management is the prevention and treatment of these secondary insults to the injured brain; and it is, therefore, essential for the doctor caring for the head-injured to be able to recognize deterioration when it occurs. In some instances, the primary injury may be relatively trivial, but the delayed development of an intracranial haematoma may put the patient's life at risk.

Pathology of primary brain injury

The primary brain injury is either **closed** or **penetrating**. In Britain, the majority of head injuries are due to blunt trauma, and penetrating head injuries are relatively rare. The latter are seen more frequently in warfare and where there is a high incidence of civil violence.

The energy of the blunt head injury dissipates through the brain causing diffuse damage, the severity and duration of which depends on the force of the blow.

The relatively minor injury resulting in a brief period of unconsciousness causes a physiological disturbance without extensive anatomical disruption. With increasing severity of injury there is anatomical disruption, with damage to axons and synapses, and small areas of haemorrhage resulting in prolonged periods of unconsciousness or death. This diffuse injury of the brain can occur without a direct impact if severe inertial forces are applied, as, for example, when the head abruptly comes to rest in the impact of a road traffic accident. The same mechanism is responsible for the damage caused when children are forcibly shaken in the course of non-accidental injury.

The kinetic energy of the moving head is abruptly transformed as the head comes to rest, and a shock wave passes through the skull and brain. A certain amount of energy may be dissipated when the skull is fractured, thus reducing the energy transmitted to the brain. Since the kinetic energy of different tissues depends on the density of the tissue the energy transfer to different structures leads to shearing forces and disruption of axons.

Blunt trauma is also capable of causing focal damage. At the site of the blow the transient deformity of the skull causes local contusion of the underlying brain, with patchy areas of haemorrhage and necrosis. This **cerebral contusion** is commonly also seen at the opposite side of the head from the site of the blow—the so-called **contre-coup** injury (Fig. 1.1). The patient who falls backwards, for instance, striking the occiput is commonly found to have contusions of the frontal lobes. As a result of the impact, the temporal lobes may be contused or frankly lacerated by the sharp edge of the sphenoid ridge anteriorly. Cerebral contusions are not static lesions, and following the injury there may be coalescence of areas of haemorrhage, and progressive swelling at the contused site may occur, giving rise to neurological deterioration.

The effect of the primary injury is recognized by the patient's state of consciousness and focal neurological deficit immediately after the impact. Thus the patient who is unconscious and has a hemiparesis at the scene of the accident is likely to have a diffuse concussional injury and a unilateral cerebral contusion. By contrast, the patient who is not unconscious, or is only briefly so, has had no significant primary injury,

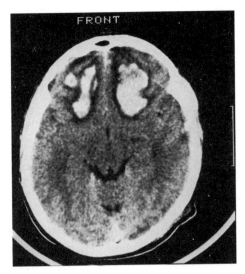

Fig. 1.1 CT scan of bifrontal cerebral contusion caused by occipital head injury—*contre-coup* injury.

and any subsequent alteration in consciousness is due to some form of potentially reversible secondary insult.

Penetrating injuries range from low-velocity injuries, with local damage to scalp and skull in the form of a depressed skull fracture and local injury to meninges and brain, to missile injuries which cause more extensive brain damage. Compound depressed skull fractures are common in civilian practice and are generally not associated with severe brain injuries. Their chief significance is that they may be complicated by infection in the form of meningitis or cerebral abscess if not recognized and treated appropriately. Gunshot injuries cause more extensive brain injuries and the severity of the damage depends on the anatomical course of the missile and its velocity. Low-velocity injuries, such as those caused by air rifles, may cause remarkably little damage unless they injure important structures in their paths. Air rifle pellets can cause devastating damage if they injure cerebral arteries. High-velocity gunshot injuries, on the other hand, are associated with severe damage to the brain beyond the track of the missile as the energy of the missile is translated into pressure waves spreading out from the track to the surrounding brain.

Intracranial pressure and cerebral perfusion

The brain occupies an inelastic container, and any increase in the volume of the contents of the skull results in a rise in pressure. Cerebral

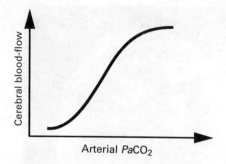

Fig. 1.2   Effect of changes in $PaCO_2$ on cerebral blood flow (CBF).

perfusion depends on two factors—cerebral perfusion pressure (CPP) and cerebrovascular resistance. Cerebral perfusion pressure depends on systemic arterial blood pressure (Fig. 1.2), while cerebrovascular resistance is determined by intracranial pressure (ICP). Cerebrovascular resistance may be increased by extracranial venous obstruction, as when the jugular veins are compressed in the neck or when venous return is impeded by tilting the patient head-down. A rise in intracranial pressure not accompanied by a rise in blood pressure leads to reduced cerebral perfusion, as expressed in the equation:

$$CPP = BP - ICP.$$

Cerebral perfusion pressure less than 40 mmHg results in a critical reduction in cerebral blood flow.

Rising pressure above the tentorium results in displacement of the brain in a caudal direction as the severity of the condition increases. The medial aspects of the temporal lobes eventually herniate through the tentorial hiatus. The upper brainstem is directly compressed, the medulla impacts in the foramen magnum, and the respiratory centre is rendered ischaemic. The herniating temporal lobe stretches the ipsilateral oculomotor nerve. Compression of the oculomotor nerve results in dilatation of the pupil, which finally fails to respond to light (Fig. 1.3).

In response to rising intracranial pressure, there is a reflex increase in systemic blood pressure and slowing of pulse rate—the Cushing reflex.

Increased intracranial pressure following head injury is caused by **diffuse swelling** or by **intracranial haematoma**, and sometimes by **cerebrospinal fluid obstruction**, or by a combination of all these factors. Swelling of the brain is due to oedema or to increase in the cerebral blood volume. $PaCO_2$ has a very important influence on intracranial pressure. The cerebral arterioles are sensitive to changes in $PaCO_2$, dilat-

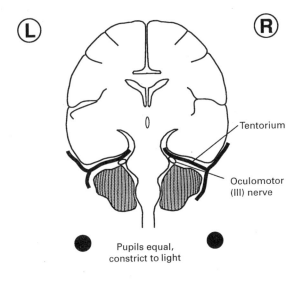

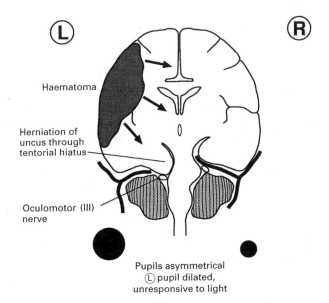

Fig. 1.3 Mechanism of tentorial herniation due to intracranial haematoma.

ing in response to a rise in $PaCO_2$ and constricting in response to a reduction in $PaCO_2$. The resulting change in intracranial blood volume leads to changes in intracranial pressure (Fig. 1.4). An increase in $PaCO_2$ from 5.3 kPa (40 mmHg) to 10.6 kPa (80 mmHg) leads to a doubling of the cerebral blood flow and a reduction from 5.3 to 2.6 kPa to a halving

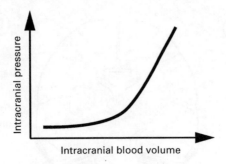

Fig. 1.4   Relation of intracranial pressure (ICP) to intracranial blood volume.

of the cerebral blood flow. A rising $PaCO_2$ due to impaired ventilation in the head-injured patient leads to a rising intracranial pressure and impaired cerebral perfusion. Conversely, lowering the $PaCO_2$ by hyperventilation brings about a reduction in intracranial pressure, and is used to this end in the intensive management of severe head injuries. The critical importance of respiratory complications in the management of the head-injured patient will be referred to in subsequent chapters.

Cerebrovascular autoregulation

The arterioles of the cerebral circulation regulate cerebral blood flow. In the healthy individual, the cerebral arterioles respond to systemic hypotension to as low as 60 mmHg by dilating and maintaining a constant cerebral blood flow. Conversely, systemic hypertension up to 160 mmHg does not result in an increase in cerebral blood flow because the cerebral arterioles constrict accordingly. This autoregulatory mechanism is impaired after injury to the brain, and a reduction in arterial blood pressure may result in decreased cerebral blood flow. The cerebral perfusion is vulnerable to fluctuations in systemic blood pressure. The treatment of shock and blood loss is therefore a priority in the management of severe head injury.

The measurement of conscious level

It is of crucial importance to those caring for head-injured patients to be able to recognize changes in conscious level. This must be done in a precise and universally accepted fashion. Terms such as 'semi-conscious' or 'comatose' are not acceptable. The internationally accepted scale of consciousness is the **Glasgow Coma Scale** (Box 1.3).

Box 1.3 Glasgow Coma Scale

		Score
Eye-opening response	Spontaneously	4
	To speech	3
	To pain	2
	Do not open	1
Best verbal response	Orientated	5
	Confused	4
	Inappropriate words	3
	Incomprehensible sounds	2
	None	1
Best motor response	Obeys commands	5
	Localizes to pain	4
	Flexes limbs to pain	3
	Extends limbs to pain	2
	None	1
Total		14

The scale is divided into three sections—the best eye-opening response, the best motor response, and the best verbal response.

Eye-opening response

Record whether the patient opens the eyes spontaneously, in response to speech, in response to pain, or not at all.

An appropriate painful stimulus is achieved by applying pressure to the supraorbital nerve or applying pressure to the ear lobe. Pressing the nail-bed is not a suitable stimulus, since this will even elicit a response in the brain dead patient, and the response, even in patients who are capable of localizing to a painful stimulus, is invariably to flex the limb.

A numerical value can be attached to each component of the scale, and the sum of the three recordings gives a Coma Score, which can be used to subdivide head-injured patients into groups according to conscious level. The maximum score in the fully conscious patient is 14.

The Glasgow Coma Scale (GCS) is one of the most important developments in the management of head injury. The GCS makes it possible to recognize changes in consciousness reflecting recovery or deterioration. It is therefore a dynamic scoring system that must be reused at regular intervals. It enables the doctor with responsibility for the head-injured patient to give a precise description of the patient's conscious level to the neurosurgeon, and it provides one means of quantifying the severity of the injury. A modification of the scale is required in young children, and this is described in Chapter 8.

Motor response

The **motor response** is recorded as obeying commands, localizing to painful stimuli, flexing the limbs in response to pain, extending the limbs, or no response. Suitable commands include 'put out your tongue' or 'hold up two fingers'. Placing the examiner's fingers in the palm of the patient's hand may elicit a grasp reflex, and give a false impression that the patient is obeying the command 'squeeze my fingers'. Some charts include a category—'withdrawal' or 'abnormal flexion'—in the motor response to pain. This addition to the original Glasgow Coma Scale is often difficult to define and poorly understood by those responsible for carrying out the recordings, and should be omitted. Purposeful movements such as pulling at the bedclothes, scratching, or attempting to remove the nasogastric tube are equivalent to localizing to a painful stimulus.

Verbal response

The **verbal response** is recorded as orientated (in place, time, and person), confused (speaking in formed sentences but not orientated), inappropriate words (often expletives!), and incomprehensible sounds. Spurious results may be obtained if the patient is dysphasic.

Further reading

Field, J. H (1976). *Epidemiology of head injuries in England and Wales.* HMSO, London.

Jennett, B. and Teasdale, G. (1981). *Management of head injuries* (Contemporary Neurology Series). F. A. Davis, Philadelphia.

Jennett, B. *et al.* (1977). Severe head injuries in three countries. *Journal of Neurology, Neurosurgery, and Psychiatry,* **40**, 291–8.

Jennett, B. *et al.* (1978). Head injuries in three Scottish neurosurgical units. *British Medical Journal,* **2**, 955–8.

2 Initial assessment

Key points in initial assessment

1 Most patients admitted to hospital after head injury are conscious and have no neurological deficit. They are admitted principally for observation, because the nature of their primary injury exposes them to delayed complications which may require prompt recognition and treatment.

2 In the unconscious patient it is vital to establish whether there has been a change in conscious level since the injury, as this may indicate a developing intracranial haematoma.

3 Severe headache and vomiting are indications for admission, as they may herald an intracranial haematoma or meningitis.

4 Any history of the consumption of alcohol or other drugs should be recorded, as should any bleeding or fluid discharge from nose or ears.

5 Absence of suitable supervision at home is an indication for observation in hospital.

6 The patient's state of alertness and conscious level should be recorded using the Glasgow Coma Scale.

7 By no means all head-injured patients require skull X-rays, and the main purpose of the skull X-ray is to determine whether the patient requires admission.

8 All patients with altered consciousness should have their blood sugar measured by the stick method.

9 The patient with a skull fracture who is not fully conscious has a 25% chance of having a haematoma of some sort. In children, 40% of extradural haematomas occur without radiological evidence of a fracture.

10 The patient with cerebrospinal fluid (CSF) rhinorrhoea or otorrhoea should be admitted until the discharge has ceased or the fistula has been repaired.

11 The patient who has had a fit following injury may have further post-traumatic fits, and should be admitted for observation.

12 In head-injured patients with an impaired conscious level who are known to be affected by alcohol one must always assume that the impairment is due to the injury, and investigate or observe the patient appropriately.

In the case of the severely injured patient, and particularly the multiply injured patient, the first priority is to carry out a rapid assessment of the airway, breathing, and circulation, and to initiate resuscitation. However, of the very large number of patients seen every year in A&E departments

Box 2.1 Facts to be established on initial assessment

- Has the patient had a head injury?
- Has the patient a scalp or skull injury requiring treatment?
- Does the patient require admission to hospital?

following head injuries the great majority do not require admission, and a majority of those who do are conscious and have no neurological deficit. These patients require to be admitted not because they have suffered a severe primary injury but because the nature of the injury exposes them to potentially serious complications. In order to recognize and treat delayed complications of the head injury promptly, these patients are admitted principally for observation. Only a minority have severe primary injuries, and the need for admission in this group is usually self-evident. The assessment and resuscitation of the patient with severe head injury is dealt with in Chapter 3.

The initial assessment, including the history, examination and investigations, should establish the facts shown in Box 2.1.

The history

The history should establish whether the patient has had a head injury. In some instances it may be clear that the patient collapsed because of some preceding loss of consciousness. It is important to establish how the injury happened. The circumstances of the injury indicate the severity of the blow, and draw attention to possible associated injuries. Where no clear history is available from the patient every effort should be made to interview relatives, ambulance crews, police, and other observers. In the case of the unconscious patient, it is particularly vital to establish whether there has been a change in conscious level since the time of the injury, indicating the possibility of a developing intracranial haematoma. If the patient was capable of talking at some stage after the injury the primary brain injury cannot have been severe. The time of the accident should be established. The greater the interval between injury and admission the greater the chance that the patient's neurological condition at the time of examination may have evolved since the impact.

A history of unconsciousness following the injury indicates that there has been a significant blow. The duration of unconsciousness should be recorded. The patient should be asked about headache and vomiting, about symptoms related to cranial nerve injuries—diplopia, facial numb-ness, facial weakness, deafness, dysarthria—and about symptoms of weakness or altered sensation in the limbs.

Severe headache and/or vomiting after a head injury are worrying symptoms, and are indications that the patient should be admitted. They may herald an intracranial haematoma or meningitis.

Note whether there has been any bleeding or discharge of fluid from the nose or ears.

Any history of the consumption of alcohol or other drugs should be recorded. The patient's altered state of consciousness may in part be due to alcohol, and evidence of alcohol consumption may be of medico-legal importance. A history of chronic alcohol abuse draws attention to the possibilities of alcohol withdrawal symptoms after admission and of impaired blood coagulation.

If the patient is to be discharged from the A&E department, it is necessary to establish whether there will be adequate supervision at home. If the patient has had a significant injury but is thought not to require admission, written instructions should be provided for the next of kin, who should be encouraged to bring the patient back if there is any cause for concern. Absence of suitable supervision at home is an indication for observation in hospital.

The examination

In head injury, as in other forms of trauma, it is important to adhere to the standard sequence of **airway**, **breathing**, and **circulation** when carrying out the initial assessment and resuscitation. These priorities must be dealt with appropriately before a more detailed examination is performed.

The scalp

Examine the scalp for evidence of trauma. These signs may be confined to small scalp abrasions or contusions. Scalp lacerations must be care-fully explored for fractures and foreign bodies; but this should be delayed until the doctor is prepared to suture the wound, since examin-ation may provoke fresh bleeding. The ear should be drawn forwards so that bruising over the mastoid bone can be seen (Battle's sign), indicating fracture of the petrous bone. Examine the ears with an otoscope for evid-ence of haemotympanum, which may be found in association with frac-tures of the petrous bone. Periorbital bruising is evidence of a fracture of the anterior cranial fossa, which may involve the cribriform plate or paranasal air sinuses. Patients with fractures of the base of the anterior fossa or the petrous bone are at risk of developing meningitis. The nose and ears should be inspected for evidence of bleeding or cerebrospinal fluid (CSF) discharge.

Vital signs

The pulse and blood pressure are recorded and are taken repeatedly at half-hourly or hourly intervals, depending on the severity of the injury, while the patient remains under observation. A variety of patterns of pulse and blood pressure is seen, depending on the severity of the injury and the extent of associated injuries.

Commonly in the unconscious patient, hypertension and tachycardia are the initial findings. Once the airway has been cleared and any injured limbs have been splinted the pulse and blood pressure may return to normal values. Hypertension with bradycardia implies raised intracranial pressure: but this is by no means always found in patients with an intracranial mass, and, when present, is often a late development. Hypotension is very rarely due to the head injury itself, and should suggest the possibility of blood loss. Hypotension may also be seen in the patient with spinal cord injury.

Conscious level

The single most important observation in the head-injured patient is the recording of conscious level. Just as pulse and blood pressure recording is crucial to the management of shock, the recording of conscious level enables the doctor to determine both the severity of the brain injury and to recognize changes in consciousness and, hence, complications of the injury and response to treatment. Vague terms such as 'unconscious' or 'semiconscious' are of no value and do not provide the baseline required to recognize subsequent changes in conscious level. The level of consciousness on arrival in hospital must be recorded in the terms of the Glasgow Coma Scale (p. 13, Box 1.3) or, in the case of a child, using the modified paediatric coma scale (p. 124, Box 8.3). The three components of the coma scale should be recorded in words. Simply recording a numerical value for the conscious level can be misleading as, for example, when the patient is dysphasic but fully conscious. The admission conscious level reflects the effect of the primary brain injury and any deterioration in consciousness indicates that some secondary injury to the brain, systemic or intracranial, is taking place.

It is very important to be aware that agitation and disturbed behaviour is a feature of altered consciousness and the head-injured patient who behaves in a violent or abusive fashion cannot be assumed simply to be drunk or malicious. Such patients have been known to die in a police cell when the effects of an intracranial haematoma were mistaken for drunk and disorderly behaviour.

Cranial nerves

Examine the cranial nerves when appropriate. Detailed examination of each cranial nerve is indicated only if circumstances suggest the possibility of a cranial nerve injury. Examination of the cranial nerves must not be neglected simply because the patient is not fully conscious. It is quite possible to examine most of the cranial nerves without the patient's cooperation. Injuries of the cranial nerves are discussed in Chapter 6.

Olfactory nerves

The sense of smell can be tested in the conscious patient by occluding one nostril and presenting any strongly scented substance to the other nostril. The patient should indicate whether the scent is apparent, and need not be able to name the substance.

Optic nerves

In the head-injured patient, the optic fundi are invariably normal in the hours immediately following the injury. Retinal haemorrhages may be seen in those patients who have collapsed as a result of spontaneous intracranial haemorrhage. It is not desirable to dilate the pupils in order to see the optic fundi, since the pupil's size and reaction to light are an important part of continuing neurological observations.

Visual acuity is measured using either the Snellen chart set at 6 metres (20 feet) from the patient or books of standard print (e.g. Jaeger charts). If the patient uses spectacles these should be worn at first one eye and then the other and tested separately.

To examine the visual fields the examiner sits facing the patient and covers one of the patient's eyes with his/her own hand. The patient is then asked to look at the examiner's pupil while an object is brought into the field of vision. A pinhead may be used as the object or, failing that, the examiner's finger. Each quadrant of the field of vision is tested in one eye and then in the other. The patient is asked to indicate when the pinhead is seen, or when a small movement of the examiner's fingertip is recognized. Visual field defects are rarely seen on initial assessment, as they usually follow severe injuries, and require the patient's cooperation.

Cranial nerves 3–6

Record the pupil sizes and their reactions to light. Dilatation of the pupil and an absent light reflex indicate a defect in either the afferent limb or the efferent limb of the light reflex. An afferent pupillary defect is due to injury of the retina or the optic nerve, whereas an efferent pupillary defect is caused by a lesion of the third (oculomotor) cranial nerve or a direct injury of the iris. Injury of the third (oculomotor) nerve may be caused by direct trauma associated with a skull base fracture, or indirectly as a result of herniation of the temporal lobe through the tentorial hiatus. In the latter case, the dilated pupil will be associated with impaired consciousness, whereas in the case of a direct injury of the eye or the nerve alone the patient will be alert, but may have other evidence of injury to the orbit.

By using the consensual reflex it is possible to demonstrate whether unilateral loss of the light reflex is due to an afferent or an efferent defect. In the case of an afferent defect, the pupil will react in response to stimulus to the other eye. In the case of an efferent defect, the pupil of the opposite eye will react in response to a light shone in the abnormal eye. Since the oculomotor nerve is also responsible for the innervation of some extraocular muscles and levator palpebrae its injury may be accompanied by a ptosis and ocular palsy.

Examine the eye movements by asking the patient to follow a moving finger. In the uncooperative patient observation alone may reveal impairment of eye movements. However, eye movements can be examined more precisely in the unconscious patient using the oculocephalic or 'doll's eye' reflex. As the patient's head is turned from side to side the reflex causes conjugate deviation of the eyes to the opposite side, and so the integrity of the oculomotor and abducent nerves can be established.

Trigeminal nerve

Facial sensation should be tested on either side using a pin. Examine the forehead, cheek, and chin on either side. Subtle degrees of trigeminal sensory impairment may be recognized by testing the corneal reflex with a piece of cotton-wool. The corneal reflex can be used to examine trigeminal nerve integrity in the unconscious patient.

Facial nerve

Facial weakness may be due to either an upper or a lower motor lesion. Upper motor-neuron facial weakness may be associated with a hemiparesis, and tends to spare the forehead. The lower motor-neuron lesion involves all the facial muscles. By inflicting a painful stimulus and observing the facial movement in response, it is possible to recognize a facial weakness in the unconscious patient.

Auditory and vestibular nerves

Deafness is not uncommon after head injuries where there has been disruption of the middle ear apparatus or fractures of the petrous bone.

The simplest technique for detecting deafness is to cover one ear and determine whether the whispered voice can be heard in the other ear. Using a tuning fork, Rinne's and Weber's tests reveal which ear is deaf and whether the deafness is neural or conductive.

Cranial nerves 9–12

The lower cranial nerves are very infrequently affected in head injuries, and their examination is required only if the patient has post-traumatic dysarthria.

The limbs

Examine the limbs for power and reflexes. Subtle degrees of limb weakness may be missed if the patient is simply asked to 'squeeze my fingers'. A mild hemiparesis can be unmasked by asking the patient to hold out the hands while closing the eyes. The weak arm will drift away from the initial position. In the unconscious patient, observation of the patient's spontaneous movements will reveal asymmetries indicating unilateral weakness. It may be significant that the unconscious patient makes purposeful movements with the left hand in preference to the right.

The spine

Palpate the entire length of the spine for tenderness and examine for bruising. Where there is suspicion of a spinal injury the limbs should be carefully examined for power and reflexes, and a careful sensory examination should be carried out, not neglecting the saddle area.

General examination

If the patient smells of alcohol record this. Finally, a general examination should be carried out, particularly in the unconscious patient, who may be harbouring multiple injuries.

Box 2.2 Indications for skull X-ray

- A history of unconsciousness
- Scalp bruising, haematoma, laceration
- A focal neurological deficit
- An impaired conscious level
- Difficulty in patient assessment due to age, alcohol, drugs, etc.
- CSF rhinorrhoea or otorrhoea
- Headache, vomitting
- Unconscious, ? head injury

Investigations

Most head-injured patients require minimal investigation. The main consideration in most is whether a skull X-ray should be carried out. Controversy has surrounded the question of who should have skull X-rays. By no means all patients seen in the A&E department after head injuries require X-rays, and the indications are given in Box 2.2. Essential skull views are the antero-posterior, the lateral, and the Townes view. Interpretation of skull X-rays is discussed in detail in Chapter 5. The main purpose of the skull X-ray is to determine whether the patient requires admission to hospital.

All patients with altered consciousness should have the blood sugar measured by the stick method. Altered consciousness may be due to insulin, oral hypoglycaemic agents, or alcohol.

Other investigations may be indicated by the circumstances of the injury. It should be remembered that injuries of the cervical spine are associated with head injuries when the accident has been a fall or a road traffic accident. Good-quality X-rays of the cervical spine must include the seventh cervical vertebra on the lateral projection. It may be necessary to pull the shoulders down while the lateral X-ray is taken in order to visualize the lower parts of the cervical spine.

Alcohol levels may be assayed in blood, breath, or saliva. A blood-alcohol level less than 2 g/litre makes it likely that altered consciousness is due to the head injury and not to alcohol consumption. It must be emphasized, however, that a high alcohol level cannot be assumed to be the reason for altered consciousness in the injured patient.

Indications for admission to hospital

The unconscious or multiply injured patient clearly requires admission. The conscious patient may require admission either because there is a scalp or skull injury which is unsuitable for outpatient treatment or because there are reasons to believe that the injury may be attended by delayed complications. The latter group of patients are admitted for observation and symptomatic relief.

The main source of anxiety in the case of the patient with a relatively mild primary injury is the possibility of extradural haemotoma. In adult patients, 80% of extradural haematomas are associated with a skull fracture–recognized either clinically or radiologically. In children, 40% of extradural haematomas occur without radiological evidence of a fracture. The presence of a skull fracture is, therefore, the most important risk factor in determining who is in danger of developing this potentially lethal complication. The absence of a fracture is less reassuring in children, and the indications for admission have to be broader.

The patient with a skull fracture who is not fully conscious has been shown to have as much as a 25% chance of having an intracranial haematoma of some sort.

In contrast, the conscious patient with no skull fracture has only a 1 in 6000 chance of developing an intracranial haematoma. Box 2.3 shows the risk of intracranial haematoma in different groups of patients.

In adults, a history of unconsciousness following the injury is not in itself an indication for admission, since it is associated with a very low incidence of intracranial haematoma. In children, however, it is prudent to observe the patient who has had an injury severe enough to cause loss of consciousness, partly because the absence of a skull fracture is a less reliable indication of the risk of intracranial haematoma, and partly because recognition of deterioration in the child is more difficult than in the adult. Even in good health the young child may be difficult to rouse

Box 2.3   Risk of intracranial haematoma after head injury

		Risk of intracranial haematoma
Orientated	No skull fracture	1 in 6000
Disorientated	No skull fracture	1 in 120
Orientated	Skull fracture	1 in 30
Disorientated	Skull fracture	1 in 4

Box 2.4   Indications for admission

- Altered conscious level
- Post-traumatic epileptic fit
- Focal neurological deficit
- Clinical or radiological evidence of skull fracture
- Severe headache or vomitting
- CSF rhinorrhoea/otorrhoea
- Extensive scalp laceration
- Inadequate supervision at home
- Child with history of unconsciousness

after the accustomed bedtime, and this tendency is more pronounced when the child is overwrought and exhausted after the drama of injury and hospital attendance.

Severe headache and vomiting may be symptoms of an intracranial haematoma in the patient who is fully conscious and exhibits no focal neurological deficit.

The patient with CSF rhinorrhoea or otorrhoea should be admitted until the discharge has ceased or the fistula has been repaired.

Extensive scalp lacerations should be repaired under general anaesthetic, and may be associated with significant blood loss.

The patient who has had a fit following injury may have further post-traumatic fits, and should be admitted for observation. There is a very small increased incidence of intracranial haematoma in association with post-traumatic fits (see Box 2.4).

Head injury associated with alcohol or drug ingestion

There is a strong association between alcohol and head injury, and the patient's clinical condition may be due to a combination of alcohol intoxication and head injury. In the case of a drowsy head-injured patient who has had a surfeit of alcohol it is not possible to predict the contribution made to the altered conscious state by alcohol. One must always assume that the patient's impaired conscious level is due to head injury, and investigate or observe the patient appropriately.

As has been mentioned earlier, the skull X-ray plays an important part in the decision to admit the head-injured patient to hospital. Very often the X-rays have to be interpreted by a relatively inexperienced doctor at a time when more experienced advice is not immediately available. A reliable history may not always be obtainable, and social circumstances may raise doubts as to how well the patient will be observed at home. The foregoing criteria for admission are only guide-lines, and the doctor on the spot must always act on the side of caution if there is any doubt about the significance of the injury.

Having decided that the patient requires admission, the next step is to ensure that any subsequent neurological deterioration is recognized early and acted upon.

Neurological observation

In most instances, the purpose of admitting the head-injured patient is to enable potential complications to be recognized at an early and treatable stage. To this end, observations should be directed towards recognizing neurological deterioration and evidence of a developing intracranial haematoma or other secondary causes of neurological impairment. Conscious level is also assessed at hourly intervals in the terms of the Glasgow Coma Scale. It is convenient to chart all the observations on a single neurological observation chart (Fig. 2.1). It is important to make sure that the medical and nursing staff understand the terms of the Coma Scale in order to avoid spurious apparent changes in conscious level.

Pulse rate, blood pressure, temperature, and respiratory rate should be recorded at hourly intervals. Bradycardia and hypertension are associated with rising intracranial pressure. The size of the pupils and their reaction to light are also recorded hourly. Dilatation of one pupil or a sluggish or absent response to light is an ominous sign, indicating a developing mass on the same side as the affected pupil. These signs develop in the late stages of rising intracranial pressure.

The patient with a moderate concussional head injury will usually tend to lie quietly with the eyes closed unless disturbed. If the patient begins to become restless, exhibiting purposeless activity, such as pulling at the bed-clothes or making ineffectual efforts to get over the cot sides, this represents a deterioration in conscious level. On no account should restless head-injured patients be sedated. This behaviour may herald the development of an intracranial haematoma, and should be investigated appropriately. In the absence of an operable intracranial lesion these patients can usually be contained by cot sides on the bed and nursing supervision.

Never sedate the restless head-injured patient

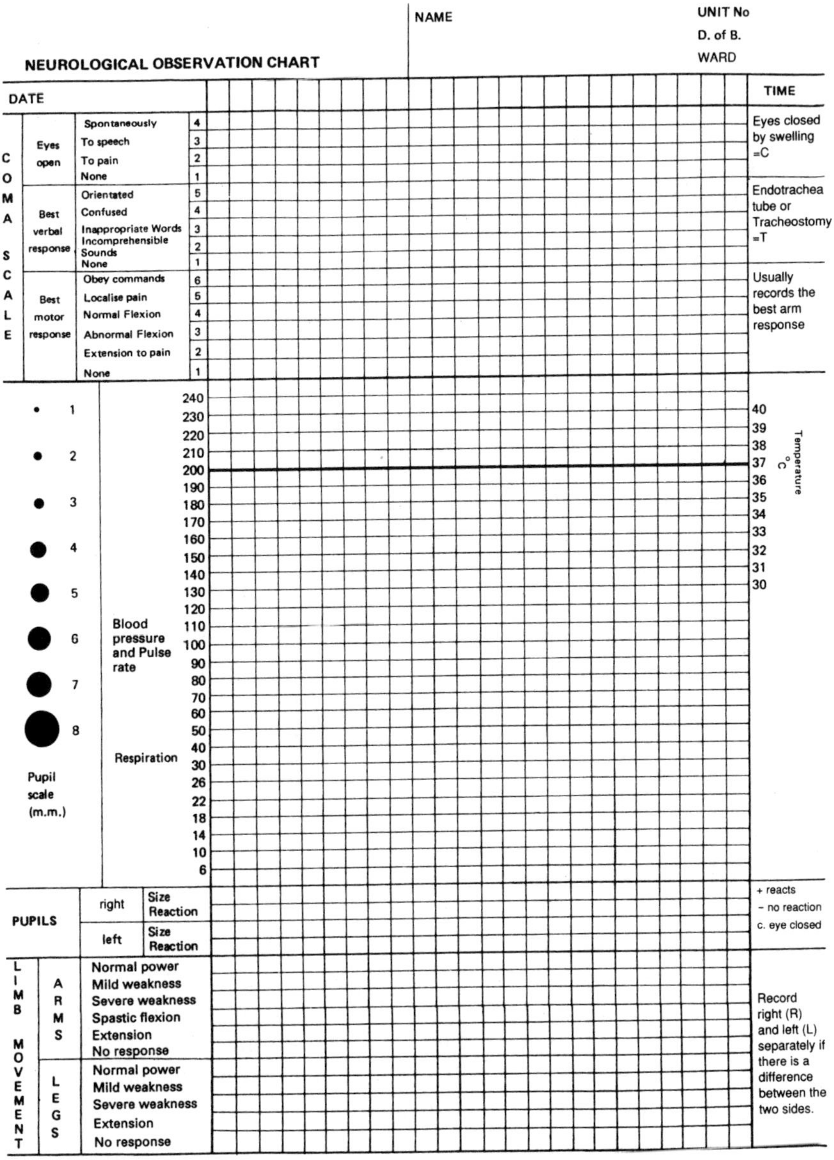

NAME

UNIT No

D. of B.

WARD

NEUROLOGICAL OBSERVATION CHART

DATE																														TIME

C O M A	Eyes open	Spontaneously	4																												Eyes closed by swelling =C
		To speech	3																												
		To pain	2																												
		None	1																												
S	Best verbal response	Orientated	5																												Endotrachea tube or Tracheostomy =T
C A		Confused	4																												
L E		Inappropriate Words	3																												
		Incomprehensible Sounds	2																												
		None	1																												
	Best motor response	Obey commands	6																												Usually records the best arm response
		Localise pain	5																												
		Normal Flexion	4																												
		Abnormal Flexion	3																												
		Extension to pain	2																												
		None	1																												

Pupil scale (m.m.)

```
• 1
• 2
• 3
● 4
● 5
● 6
● 7
● 8
```

Blood pressure and Pulse rate

Respiration

```
240
230
220
210
200
190
180
170
160
150
140
130
120
110
100
90
80
70
60
50
40
30
26
22
18
14
10
6
```

Temperature °C

```
40
39
38
37
36
35
34
33
32
31
30
```

PUPILS	right	Size																													+ reacts − no reaction c. eye closed
		Reaction																													
	left	Size																													
		Reaction																													

L I M B	A R M S	Normal power																													Record right (R) and left (L) separately if there is a difference between the two sides.
		Mild weakness																													
		Severe weakness																													
		Spastic flexion																													
M O V E M E N T		Extension																													
		No response																													
	L E G S	Normal power																													
		Mild weakness																													
		Severe weakness																													
		Extension																													
		No response																													

Fig. 2.1   A neurological observation chart (Aberdeen hospitals central nervous system — CNS — observation chart).

If it is clear after 12 to 24 hours that the patient is steadily improving the frequency of the recordings may be reduced. Most head-injured patients will need observation for approximately 24 hours, by which time there is little likelihood of delayed deterioration, and the patient may

Box 2.5   Head-injury instructions

Seek further medical advice in the event of:
- Severe headache
- Frequent vomitting
- Discharge of fluid from nose or ears
- Confusion or inappropriate drowsiness

be discharged as soon as symptoms such as headache or vomiting allow.

Patients should be discharged to the care of a responsible adult who has been given advice about simple head-injury observation and when to seek further medical attention (see Box 2.5). Relatives should not be asked to carry out formal hourly observations—particularly through the night. If this level of observation is really required the patient should be admitted to hospital rather than being sent home. Friends or relatives should be advised to bring the patient back to hospital if there is severe headache, persistent vomiting, confusion, or drowsiness. The patient should be advised to report any discharge of watery fluid from the nose or ears.

Relief of symptoms

Analgesics are required for headache, but strong opioid analgesics should be avoided, particularly in the drowsy or confused patient. Simple oral analgesics such as paracetamol or codeine phosphate are suitable for relatively minor pain. Non-steroidal antiinflammatory agents such as diclofenac are also effective, and the latter can be administered orally, intramuscularly, or in suppository form. The conscious patient with more severe pain must be given effective analgesia, and this can be achieved using reversible opioids such as morphine or papaveretum (Omnopon) intravenously, titrated to the patient's response while concern about possible intracranial complications persists. Local anaesthetic blocks may be used in some instances for relief of limb pain if narcotic analgesics are to be avoided; such blocks are most effective in the patient with a head injury complicated by a solitary limb injury.

Nausea and vomiting can be controlled with any of the standard antiemetic agents.

Outpatient review

Of the patients seen in A&E departments and either discharged or admitted for observation, only a small number should be reviewed, and most of these should be seen in the relevant specialist departments. Patients with cranial nerve injuries must be reviewed in neurosurgery, ENT (ear, nose, throat), or ophthalmology clinics as appropriate. Patients with post-traumatic epilepsy, if not already under the care of a neurosurgeon, should be reviewed in a neurosurgical clinic. Post-concussional symptoms are dealt with in most instances by general practitioners, and only occasionally require specialist referral.

Patients with uncomplicated head injuries do not require routine review in the A&E department.

Further reading

Bickerstaff, E. R. and Spillane, J. (1996). *Neurological examination in clinical practice, sixth edition.* Blackwell Scientific, Oxford.

Jennett, B. and Teasdale, G. (1981). *Management of head injuries*, (Contemporary Neurology Series). F. A. Davis, Philadelphia.

Tyson, G. W. (1987). *Head injury management for providers of emergency care.* Williams & Wilkins, Baltimore.

3 Resuscitation

Chapter contents

Key points in resuscitation

1 Resuscitation of the head-injured patient is the responsibility of the A&E department, and on no account should a patient be transferred to a specialist unit before resuscitation is complete and the patient stabilized. Hypotension and hypoxia on arrival at Neurosurgery are associated with very high mortality rates. Patients should not be removed from the resuscitation room (e. g. for X-rays) until resuscitation is complete: this may necessitate the use of portable X-ray equipment.

2 Until it is proved otherwise, patients should be assumed to have associated cervical spine injuries, and up to that point the neck should be immobilized with a rigid collar or between sandbags, and a senior member of the team should be in charge of the head and neck whenever a patient is moved.

3 Opioid analgesics and benzodiazepines should be administered with great care, and only when facilities to reverse their effects and to ventilate the patient are available, because of their respiratory depressant action.

4 Gaining control of the airway and ventilation is vital in controlling intracranial pressure and hypoxia, and failure in this can render any direct management of the head injury futile: the A&E doctor should never hesitate to ventilate in advance of a neurosurgical opinion if respiration is inadequate.

5 When deciding to use positive pressure ventilation care must be taken to exclude or to treat a pneumothorax first.

6 Endotracheal intubation and controlled ventilation should be instituted by an anaesthetist or a doctor experienced in anaesthetic technique, with an assistant applying pressure to the cricoid cartilage to prevent regurgitation of gastric contents.

7 $PaCO_2$ should be maintained between 3.5 and 4.0 kPa.

8 A computerized tomography (CT) scan is mandatory in the patient whose conscious level is deteriorating; in the patient who remains unconscious after resuscitation and in the patient with a skull fracture who is not fully conscious.

9 Anaesthetic techniques used for the treatment of other injuries must avoid exacerbating raised intracranial pressure.

10 Pain causes increased intracranial pressure in the head-injured, but opioid analgesics, including codeine, depress consciousness and respiration even in small doses, and so if used they should be given in small intravenous aliquots under close observation.

Priorities in resuscitation

Resuscitation of the head-injured patient is the responsibility of the staff in the A&E department, and the outcome of the injury depends crucially on the effectiveness of this early stage in the patient's treatment. It cannot be stressed too often that general resuscitation must precede all other considerations.

The management of severe head injuries is governed by the same principles as that of other forms of trauma—**Airway, Breathing**, and **Circulation**, in that order of priority. It is easy to be distracted by the apparent severity of the head injury, especially, for example, when there is a major compound injury; but the successful management of the head injury depends first and foremost on the effectiveness of the general resuscitation. On no account should the head-injured patient be transferred to a specialist unit before resuscitative measures have been completed and the patient's condition has been stabilized. (See Box 3.1.)

Head-injury resuscitation is the responsibility of the doctor in A&E department

---

A study in Glasgow in 1981 by Gentleman and Jennett illustrated the influence of extracranial injuries on the outcome after head injury. Patients with hypotension and/or hypoxia were compared with those with neither complication. Patients who were hypotensive on arrival in the neurosurgical unit had a mortality rate of 75%, and those who were hypoxic a mortality rate of 59%. There were no survivors in the group who had been both hypotensive and hypoxic. This was compared with a 34% mortality in those patients who had suffered neither insult. A study by Kohi and Mendelow in 1984 showed similarly unfavourable results

Box 3.1   Priorities in resuscitation

- Stabilize cervical spine
- Airway
- Breathing
- Circulation
- Neurological assessment

when the quality of outcome in surviving patients was related to the occurrence of hypotension and hypoxia.

Clinical assessment, resuscitation, and investigation must be conducted simultaneously in the resuscitation room. Appropriate early investigations are those that will contribute directly to the process of resuscitation. In general, the patient should not be moved from the resuscitation room (e. g. for X-rays) until resuscitation is complete. This may require X-rays of the chest, cervical spine, or pelvis to be performed using portable equipment. X-rays of minor limb injuries or obvious fractures are not required until resuscitation has been completed.

Cervical spine

Until it is proved otherwise, head-injured patients arriving in the A&E department should be assumed to have an associated spinal injury. Until this has been assessed clinically and radiologically, the neck should be immobilized, either with a rigid collar or, in the case of the deeply unconscious patient, between sandbags. Care must be exercised when moving the patient (e.g. from the ambulance trolley to the A&E trolley). A senior member of the team should be in charge of stabilizing the head and neck whenever it is necessary to lift the patient from one surface to another.

Airway and breathing

Respiratory insufficiency commonly accompanies head injury, and constitutes the most important cause of avoidable morbidity and mortality. Respiratory insufficiency is due either to **central factors** or to **peripheral factors**.

Central respiratory impairment

The unconscious patient readily obstructs the upper airway because of the tendency of the tongue to fall back and occlude the oropharynx. Loss of the protective airway reflexes exposes the patient to the risk of vomiting and aspirating gastric contents. Abnormal patterns of respiration are seen in the unconscious head-injured patient; but respiratory depression directly due to the brain injury itself is rare, except as a terminal event. Central depression of respiration is more commonly due to the effects of alcohol, drugs, or epileptic fits. Opioid analgesics and benzodiazepines are potent respiratory depressants in the head-injured patient, and should

Box 3.2   Causes of respiratory impairment

Central causes	● Drugs
	● Brainstem injury
Peripheral causes	● Airway obstruction
	● Aspiration of blood/vomit
	● Chest trauma
	● Adult respiratory distress syndrome
	● Pulmonary oedema

be administered with great care, and only when facilities are available to reverse their effects and to ventilate the patient. Epileptic fits, due to either the primary brain injury, hypoxia, or a known previous epileptic condition, will cause respiratory insufficiency. Most fits are self-limiting; but prolonged fits (status epilepticus) or recurrent fits require treatment, partly because of respiratory considerations. All the drugs used to treat status epilepticus can cause respiratory depression, and must be used with appropriate caution. (See Box 3.2.)

Peripheral respiratory impairment

Upper airway obstruction may be caused by blood, teeth, or dentures, or by fractures of the facial skeleton. Fractures of the facial skeleton cause respiratory impairment either because of severe associated haemorrhage or because the posterior displacement of the face itself occludes the oropharynx. The severe impacted facial fracture is recognized by a 'dish-faced' deformity and by bilateral periorbital haematomas. Fractures of the mandible may also be associated with respiratory obstruction, particularly if bilateral fractures exist and the patient is lying horizontally in the supine position.

   Chest and head injuries commonly coexist in the same patient. Inspection will reveal contusions of the chest wall, asymmetrical expansion, and paradoxical movement. Surgical emphysema indicates the presence of a pneumothorax. An early chest x-ray is an essential part of the process of resuscitation. The chest X-ray may show rib fractures, pulmonary contusion, and pneumothorax. The latter may not be obvious on the supine chest X-ray, which should be repeated if there is clinical evidence of respiratory impairment. Similarly, pulmonary contusion may not be obvious on an early X-ray, and after the passage of an hour or two a further X-ray can show an alarming change in a contused lung.

'Neurogenic' pulmonary oedema sometimes occurs as a result of severe brain injuries, and is often resistant to diuretic therapy. Because early correction of respiratory impairment is so critically important it is not sufficient to treat pulmonary oedema with diuretics alone, and positive pressure ventilation is essential.

Adult respiratory distress syndrome, fat embolus, and chest infection are complications that present after the period of initial resuscitation, and are discussed in Chapter 4.

Impairment ventilation has a very important bearing on the outcome of the head injury. First, the already injured brain can ill tolerate the additional insult of hypoxia, and the conscious level may deteriorate dramatically as a result. Second, the arterial $PaCO_2$ has an important direct effect on intracranial pressure. Cerebral arterioles dilate in response to a rise in $PaCO_2$, with a consequent increase in cerebral blood flow and intracranial blood volume, and intracranial pressure is elevated. Since intracranial pressure may already be critically elevated by brain swelling or intracranial haemorrhage, every effort must be made to avoid any further exacerbation. These effects are immediate and require urgent action. Hence, gaining control of the airway and ventilation is absolutely vital. Failure to do so renders any effort directed towards direct management of the head injury futile. This is so important that **the doctor in the A&E department should never be deterred from proceeding to ventilate the patient in advance of a neurosurgical opinion if the patient's respiration is inadequate**.

Airway management

Management of the airway begins with the removal of any upper airway obstruction. This is done under direct vision with the aid of a laryngoscope, McGill forceps, and a Yankauer sucker. The mouth and pharynx must be cleared of teeth, blood, and vomit. The airway should then be kept patent by preventing obstruction by the tongue. The examiner's fingers are placed behind the angles of the mandibles and the mandible is drawn forwards—the 'jaw thrust' manoeuvre. A Guedel oral airway should be inserted. The patient who will not tolerate an oral airway should be nursed in the lateral ('recovery') position once resuscitation is complete. Bleeding from facial fractures can be torrential, and may in its own right make endotracheal intubation necessary in order to protect the airway.

Intubation and ventilation

The head-injured patient who has inadequate respiration requires intubation and positive-pressure ventilation as a matter of priority. Ventilation

Box 3.3 Indications for intubation and ventilation

- Upper airway obstruction
- Coma (GCS < 8)
- Loss of protective reflexes
- Inadequate ventilation
  - $PaO_2 < 9$ kPa on air
  - $PaO_2 < 13$ kPa on oxygen
  - $PaCO_2 > 6$ kPa
- Tachypnoea causing $PaCO_2 < 3.5$ kPa
- Irregular respiration
- Restlessness preventing investigation and treatment

Prior to transfer

- Deterioration in conscious level
- Bilateral fractured mandible/severe facial injury
- Epileptic seizures
- Severe multiple injuries

is indicated for the reasons listed in Box 3.3. It may be impossible to maintain a clear upper airway simply by using an oral airway. Chest wall or pulmonary injury may result in impaired gas exchange, with inadequate PaO_2 and elevated $PaCO_2$ when the patient is breathing spontaneously. When deciding to use positive pressure ventilation care must be taken to exclude a pneumothorax, or to treat it by tube thoracostomy if one is present. Flail segments should be obvious on direct inspection, but a pneumothorax may not be so easily recognized, and positive pressure ventilation will exacerbate the problem if the pneumothorax is not drained. When a significant chest injury is found it is likely that, sooner or later, respiratory efficiency will deteriorate, and the patient's neurological condition with it. The PaO_2 should not be allowed to fall below 10.5 kPa (80 mmHg).

If endotracheal intubation and controlled ventilation are indicated, these procedures should be carried out by an anaesthetist or a doctor very

The head-injured patient who is not breathing effectively requires urgent ventilation

experienced in anaesthetic technique, using an induction agent such as thiopentone, propofol, or etomidate and a short-acting paralysing agent.

During intubation, an assistant should apply pressure to the cricoid cartilage (Sellick's manoeuvre) in order to prevent regurgitation of gastric contents. The 'crash' intubation by an inexperienced doctor in a struggling patient exacerbates an already raised intracranial pressure, and may be extremely damaging.

Chest X-rays and arterial blood gas readings must be taken again once the patient has been intubated and controlled ventilation has been established. (See Box 3.4.)

Arterial blood gases should be analyzed regularly during resuscitation. Correction of hypoxia may make a dramatic difference to the conscious level. Hypoxia may not be clinically obvious in the young, previously fit patient, and may only be revealed by blood gas analysis.

Having decided to ventilate the patient it is important to ensure that paralysis and sedation are maintained. This is achieved by the use of a sedative agent and a long-acting neuromuscular blocking agent given intermittently or by continuous infusion. If the patient is allowed to become 'light' and struggles against the ventilator intracranial pressure will be increased.

The adequacy of ventilation must be monitored continuously after the initial resuscitation. Following the phase of initial resuscitation, respiratory impairment remains a common cause of neurological deterioration.

Intermittent positive pressure ventilation not only ensures that respiration is supported, but can be used to reduce the intracranial pressure by lowering the $PaCO_2$. The $PaCO_2$ should be maintained between 3.5 and 4.0 kPa. $PaCO_2$ below 3 kPa causes a degree of cerebral vasoconstriction which may cause cerebral ischaemia. It is particularly important to control the $PaCO_2$ in the case of the deteriorating patient who is suspected of harbouring an intracranial haematoma. Controlled ventilation

Box 3.4   Early investigations

- Chest X-ray
- Arterial blood gases
- X-ray of cervical spine
- X-ray of pelvis
- Cross-matching of blood
- Skull X-rays
- Blood alcohol

reduces the intracranial pressure and allows time to transfer the patient, arrange the CT scan, or prepare the operating theatre. Ventilation as part of the subsequent management of the severe brain injury is discussed in Chapter 4.

In general, the more extensive the injuries in the multiply injured patient the greater the indication for intubation and ventilation.

Circulation and blood volume

The physiological mechanism of cerebrovascular auto-regulation ensures that cerebal blood flow remains constant despite fluctuations in systemic blood pressure. This mechanism is impaired following head injury, and cerebral perfusion is at the mercy of the systemic blood pressure. Consequently, blood loss and hypotension have a serious impact on cerebral perfusion. Moreover, cerebral perfusion may already be compromised by elevated intracranial pressure. As far as the head injury is concerned, then, it is an urgent matter to recognize circulatory impairment due to blood loss or reduced cardiac output.

The physiological response to raised intracranial pressure includes a rise in blood pressure and a slowing of pulse rate (the 'Cushing reflex'). This may have the effect of masking shock, and it is necessary to recognize that 'shock' in the head-injured patient has different parameters from shock in other individuals. If the patient with a severe head injury has a systolic blood pressure of 100–110 mmHg and a pulse rate of 100/minute it is likely that there is concealed extracranial haemorrhage.

It is essential that blood volume is restored and haemorrhage is arrested before consideration is given to any form of neurosurgical intervention. There is no value in operative neurosurgical intervention if the brain is not being perfused.

Serious blood loss from the head injury alone is uncommon, except in the same of small children, and other sources should be sought. Serious head injuries are commonly associated with injuries of the chest, abdomen, pelvis, and limbs, and the treatment of continuing haemorrhage from one of these sources takes priority over cranial surgery and neurological investigations such as CT scan. It may be appropriate, for

---

Blood loss and hypotension further exacerbate impaired cerebral perfusion

instance, to take the patient to the operating theatre for a splenectomy first, and, having gained control of the blood loss, then turn one's attention to the neurological problem.

Head-down tilting, for the purpose, for instance, of inserting a central venous catheter, should be avoided, since this leads to a further rise in intracranial pressure, and can lead to neurological deterioration.

Nasogastric intubation and urinary catheterization

Nasogastric intubation in the unconscious patient may be desirable in certain circumstances, such as in the case of associated abdominal injuries or in the patient who is thought to have a full stomach. There are hazards in passing a nasogastric tube, however. The procedure may induce retching or vomiting, with potential ill effects on the head injury through raising the intracranial pressure. Great care should be exercised in passing nasogastric tube in the patient with major skull base fractures, as there is a risk that the tube will pass through the fracture into the cranial cavity. In such cases, orogastric intubation should be performed.

Catheterization of the bladder may be desirable in the case of severe multiple injuries with hypotension; but it is not necessary in the management of the patient who has only sustained a head injury. The unconscious patient will void urine perfectly satisfactorily, and, in the male, a urinary sheath will often suffice. The unconscious female patient will require a urinary catheter.

Other injuries

Cervical spine fractures are commonly associated with head injuries, and in the initial period after admission there is a considerable risk that further damage may be inflicted during intubation and transfer from trolley to X-ray couch and bed. Throughout the period of resuscitation the possibility of a cervical spine injury should be remembered, and the head and neck should be controlled whenever the patient is moved. The conscious patient will complain of neck pain in the presence of a spinal injury; but the unconscious patient must be treated as if the cervical spine has been injured until it is proved otherwise. A full-length lateral X-ray of the cervical spine, and an antero-posterior view showing the odontoid process are required. If a cervical fracture or subluxation is suspected the neck should be splinted in a rigid collar; but care must be taken to ensure that this is not applied so tightly that cerebral venous return is obstructed.

Other injuries may demand early attention; but it is necessary at this stage, having stabilized respiration and blood volume, to assess the patient's neurological condition.

Neurological assessment

The most important aspect of the neurological assessment is to determine whether and how the patient's conscious level is changing. The severity of the initial brain injury is reflected by the patient's conscious level at the time of injury and after resuscitation. The management of this primary brain injury amounts to providing a suitable physiological environment in which to enable spontaneous recovery to take place. A minority of patients will have a progressive neurological condition due to intracranial haemorrhage, and this is recognized by a deterioration in conscious level following the initial impact.

Conscious level may be affected by systemic factors described above (hypotension, hypoxia), and it is necessary to record the patient's conscious level after resuscitation has been affected. Regular conscious level recordings are then carried out along with measurements of pulse rate, blood pressure, respiratory rate, and temperature. Any deterioration in conscious level from this point is an indication of some secondary brain injury, as outlined in Chapter 4.

As part of the neurological examination, the scalp should be carefully examined for external evidence of injury. Penetrating head injuries may be hidden by hair unless the scalp is closely inspected. Bruising over the mastoid process and periorbital haematomas are noted as evidence of skull base injury. Examine the ears and nose for evidence of cerebrospinal fluid (CSF) leakage. The pupil size and responsiveness to light are recorded, as are focal neurological deficits. Limb weakness may only be recognized by observing the patient's spontaneous movements or responses to painful stimuli. (See Box 3.5.)

Box 3.5   Neurological assessment

- Conscious level (Glasgow Coma Scale)
- Pupil size and light reflex
- Scalp injuries
- CSF otorrhoea/rhinorrhoea
- Limb weakness

At this stage, skull X-rays should be carried out, since the presence of a skull fracture is an important risk factor in the recognition of extradural haematoma.

Indications for CT scanning

Following resuscitation and the establishment of a neurological baseline, consideration should be given to whether further neurological investigations are required. The criteria for CT scanning are detailed in Box 3.6, but it must be emphasized that a CT scan is mandatory in the patient whose conscious level is deteriorating and in the patient who remains unconscious after resuscitation, with a Glasgow Coma Score of 8 or less. A scan is also indicated in the patient with a skull fracture who is not fully conscious, since this combination of factors is associated with a 25% incidence some sort of intracranial haematoma on CT scanning.

If it is necessary to ventilate the patient for any reason it is no longer possible to monitor conscious level, and a CT scan is necessary in order to exclude an operable intracranial haemotoma. A scan is also indicated if it is necessary to anaesthetize the patient for long orthopaedic procedures during which no neurological observations are possible.

Box 3.6   Criteria for CT scan

- Patient remains unconscious after resuscitation
- Patient with depressed conscious level and skull fracture
- Patient with depressed conscious level and focal deficit
- Patient with skull fracture and focal deficit
- Patient with deteriorating conscious level
- Patient with head injury who requires ventilation
- Patient with head injury who requires general anaesthetic for orthopaedic surgery

After resuscitation and the initial neurological assessment, it may be necessary to proceed to surgical treatment of other injuries. Compound fractures and abdominal injuries often require early treatment, and it is well established that major limb fractures are best treated and stabilized early. Great care must be taken to avoid exacerbating the brain injury during this period. Inappropriate anaesthetic techniques causing hypoxia, hypercapnia, or raised intracranial pressure, together with hypotension, can be responsible for further neurological damage. The patient should be treated by an experienced anaesthetist.

Anaesthetic technique must avoid exacerbating raised intracranial pressure

---

Analgesia

The choice of analgesic for the multiply injured patient often causes anxiety. The control of pain is important not only for humanitarian reasons but also because pain causes increased intracranial pressure in the head-injured patient. Opioid analgesics, including codeine, cause depression of consciousness and respiration, and may do so in small doses in the head-injured patient. If they are used they should be administered in small intravenous aliquots, and the patient must be closely observed. The choice of analgesic techniques is discussed in Chapter 2 p. 28.

The management of a patient whose conscious level is deteriorating is discussed in the next chapter.

Further reading

Doris, P. E. and Wilson, R. A. (1985). The next logical step in the emergency radiographic evaluation of cervical spine trauma: The five view trauma series. *Journal of Emergency Medicine*, **3**, 371–5.

Frost, E. (1977). Respiratory problems associated with head trauma. *Neurosurgery*, **1**, 300–5.

Gentleman, D. and Jennett, B. (1981). Hazards of inter-hospital transfer of comatose head-injured patients. *Lancet*, **2**, 853–5.

Jennett, B. and Teasdale, G. (1981). *Management of head injuries* (Contemporary Neurology Series), (chapter 9). F. A. Davies, Philadelphia.

Kohi, Y. M. Mendelow, A. W. *et al.* (1984). Extracranial insults and outcome in patients with acute head injury—relationship to the Glasgow Coma Scale. *Injury*, **16**, 25–9.

Miller, J. D. (1978). Early insults to the injured brain. *Journal of the American Medical Association*, **240**, 439–42.

4 *Neurological deterioration*

Chapter contents

Key points in neurological deterioration

1 A very large part of the time and effort spent in the care of head-injured patients is applied to recognizing secondary brain injury.
2 After general resuscitation, simple remediable causes of deterioration should be excluded before considering transfer to a neuro-surgical unit and computerized tomographic (CT) scanning.
3 The commonest of these causes is impaired respiration—hypoxia, or CO_2 retention causing increased intracranial pressure.
4 Impaired respiration is most frequently caused by facial injuries, usually leading to haemorrhage and aspiration of blood; and chest injuries leading to physical difficulties in respiration, and may be delayed in onset until after the early stages of assessment, being eventually precipitated by exhaustion: intubation and ventilation should be considered at an early stage.
5 Once patients have been ventilated a CT scan should be carried out, and transfer to a neurosurgical unit should take place, as clinical monitoring of the neurological condition is no longer possible.
6 If an epileptic fit persists for more than 2–3 minutes it should be arrested with diazepam or chlormethiazole; but these should only be used when facilities are available to ventilate the patient in the event of respiratory arrest, because of their respiratory depressant effects.
7 Where, because of unconsciousness or multiple injuries, anti-convulsants have to be given parenterally to control recurrences of fitting, only phenytoin, sodium valproate, and phenobarbitone can frequently be used: but sodium valproate should not be used in women of child-bearing age, because of its teratogenicity; and patients should have blood pressure and electrocardiogram (ECG) monitoring when phenytoin is administered, because it can cause cardiac arrhythmias and hypotension.
8 Intracranial haematoma should be treated operatively, normally in a neurosurgical unit, and where possible after a CT scan. Intracranial pressure can be temporarily reduced (1–2 hours) by intravenous diuretics such as mannitol or fusemide (not to be given to hypo-volaemic patients) to facilitate investigations or treatment.
9 The deteriorating patient with an intracranial haematoma should be anaesthetized, paralyzed, and ventilated—this is essential for long-distance inter-hospital transfer.
10 An extradural haematoma cannot be treated through a burr hole: ideally, a craniotomy is required, or failing that a burr hole extended to form a craniectomy.

The effect and outcome of a head injury depends principally on the severity of the initial impact and the extent of the damage thereby caused to the brain. This is the **primary brain injury**, the clinical results of which may range from a brief period of unconsciousness on the one hand, to prolonged coma on the other. The pathological effects of the primary injury are discussed in Chapter 1. The clinical effect of primary brain injury is recognized by the patient's conscious level and the presence and severity of neurological deficits immediately after the impact. If, for example, the patient is capable of speaking after the head injury, it is clear that the initial damage to the brain has been relatively slight, and one would expect such a patient to survive the injury if appropriately cared for. The Glasgow school of neurosurgery has coined the term **'patients who talk and die'** to highlight the fact that the patient who is capable of talking after the injury is expected to survive, unless some secondary and avoidable injury is allowed to develop unchecked. On the other hand, the patient who is only extending the limbs in response to a painful stimulus, and whose pupils fail to react to light in the immediate aftermath of the injury has suffered a severe primary injury of the brain, from which complete recovery is much less likely.

Surgical treatment of the primary injury is directed mainly at the repair of scalp and skull injuries and penetrating injuries of the brain. Treatment of the primary brain injury is supportive—the care of the unconscious patient and the prevention of further damage.

Whether the head injury is apparently minor or very severe a number of factors may complicate the injury and cause further insult to the established brain injury. This **secondary brain injury** can be anticipated and avoided or recognized and treated. The secondary injury may further exacerbate a severe primary injury, in which case treatment of the cause of deterioration is expected to restore the patient only to the state determined by the primary injury. In some instances, however, the secondary injury may complicate a relatively minor primary injury which, in itself, poses little threat to the patient. In this case, there is a danger that a patient with a relatively minor injury might die or be disabled by entirely avoidable or treatable factors.

A very large part, therefore, of the effort and time spent in the care of head-injured patients is applied to the task of recognizing the potential secondary brain injury.

The prevention of secondary brain damage depends first on recognizing the risk factors for the various complications of head injury described below, and second on ensuring that deterioration is recognized when it does occur. This, in turn, depends on the correct selection of patients for admission and on the effectiveness of head-injury observations.

Causes of deteriorating conscious level

A number of factors may cause deterioration in conscious level following a head injury (Box 4.1). All act directly or indirectly by impairing either cerebral perfusion or the delivery of oxygen to the brain. Intracranial haemorrhage is a well-known complication of head injury, causing secondary deterioration; but before jumping to the conclusion that the patient requires immediate transfer and CT scanning it is advisable first to investigate the more immediately remediable causes of deterioration. Indeed, if these systemic complications are not treated promptly the ensuing secondary brain damage may render the question of operative neurosurgical intervention academic. This means that the doctor in the A&E department or the isolated district general hospital must resist the urge to transfer the deteriorating head-injured patient to a neurosurgical unit until general resuscitative measures have been carried out and straightforward remediable causes of deterioration have been excluded.

Respiratory complications

Impaired respiration is the commonest cause of deteriorating conscious level in the head-injured patient. The injured brain is exquisitely sensitive to **hypoxia**, and the resulting deterioration in conscious level itself will

Box 4.1   Causes of deteriorating conscious level

● **Respiratory impairment**	– hypoxia
	– hypercapnia
● **Hypovolaemia**	– blood loss
	– reduced cardiac output
● **Obstructed cerebral**	– head-down tilt
venous return	– forcible intubation
	– cervical collars
● **Fits**	
● **Intracranial haematoma**	
	– extradural haematoma
	– subdural haematoma
	– intracerebral haematoma
● **Fluid overload**	– hyponatraemia
● **Drugs**	– analgesics
	– sedatives

lead to failure to maintain a clear airway and a vicious circle of respiratory impairment.

CO_2 retention causes cerebral vasodilatation, with a consequent rise in intracranial pressure. Added to an already raised pressure due to swelling of the injured brain, the effect of CO_2 retention may be to cause serious deterioration in conscious level. This effect of impaired respiration is immediate, and requires a rapid response.

It is possible to anticipate delayed respiratory impairment when the initial assessment of the patient is carried out. The chief culprits in the early stages after injury are facial and chest injuries. The former can cause upper airway obstruction when there is posterior displacement of the facial skeleton, but more frequently result in haemorrhage and aspiration of blood. Chest injuries may result in respiratory impairment as a result of pain that inhibits chest expansion, pulmonary contusion, pneumothorax, or flail chest deformity. In the early stages of assessment the patient may appear to cope with these injuries and maintain reasonable respiratory efficiency. Deterioration may be prevented by the use of oxygen by face mask, appropriate analgesia, and insertion of an intercostal chest drain where indicated. However, as exhaustion supervenes, respiratory efforts decrease. It is preferable to anticipate this development; and in the presence of such injuries one should seriously consider paralysing, intubating, and ventilating the patient at an early stage.

Early chest X-ray appearances can be deceptively normal; but after as little as one hour there can be dramatic changes, with the appearance of pneumothorax or contusional changes. Hypoxia and hypercapnia are often underestimated, and are difficult to detect clinically. In the event of a deterioration in conscious level exclude upper airway obstruction before going on to repeat the chest X-ray and arterial blood gas analysis.

Check arterial blood gases

Once the cause of respiratory impairment has been identified simple measures, such as chest physiotherapy and oxygen by face mask, or the insertion of a chest drain may be adequate to correct the patient's arterial blood gases; but, if not, early consideration should be given to artificial ventilation. The head-injured patient who is not breathing effectively must be ventilated as a matter of priority. This is nowhere more vital than when it is proposed to transfer the patient to another hospital. The decision to paralyze and ventilate a head-injured patient in respiratory difficulties should certainly not be postponed until a neurosurgical opinion has been obtained.

The head-injured patient who is not breathing effectively must be ventilated

---

Once a patient has been paralyzed and ventilated a CT scan should be performed, if this has not already been done, in order to identify any possible intracranial haematoma, since further clinical monitoring of the neurological condition is no longer possible. Thereafter, the only means of following the progress of the head injury in these patients is to monitor the intracranial pressure. These requirements make it necessary for all such patients to be admitted to a neurosurgical unit.

Delayed neurological deterioration may occur after an interval of days or week as a result of respiratory complications. Since this presents, in many instances, at a stage when the threat of intracranial haemorrhage has receded, the urge to obtain an urgent CT scan should be resisted until respiratory complications have been excluded. The unconscious or ventilated patient may develop atelectasis or lobar collapse. Without careful chest physiotherapy these developments lead to bronchopnuemonia.

The multiply injured patient is at risk of developing the **adult respiratory distress syndrome (ARDS)**—commonly 2–4 days after injury. Many factors may contribute to this condition, including shock, over-transfusion with crystalloid fluids, sepsis, chest injury, and aspiration of vomit.

Fat embolus, complicating skeletal injuries, also develops after days or weeks, but characteristically between 24 and 48 hours after injury. The first manifestation of this syndrome may be deteriorating conscious level or epileptic fits. The characteristic physical signs of fat embolus should be sought, and the arterial blood gases should be analyzed. Oxygen therapy may be sufficient to improve the conscious level; but sometimes positive pressure ventilation will be required. This condition occurs most commonly in the young victims of multiple trauma, and the potential consequences for the brain injury are grave. Ideally, patients with this combination of problems should be observed in an intensive care unit, so that prompt action is taken in the event of failing respiratory efficiency.

Ventilation must continue until the respiratory complications have resolved. This will be judged by serial chest X-rays and arterial blood gas analysis, and by the nature and quantity of tracheal secretions.

Blood volume depletion

Hypotension due either to blood loss or to impaired cardiac output leads to further impairment of cerebral perfusion. A deterioration in conscious level after head injury may be due to continuing blood loss from a variety of sources. Remember that the parameters for shock must be reset in the patient with severe head injury (Chapter 3). Hypotension is rarely due to the head injury itself, unless there has been a very major scalp laceration.

Raised intracranial pressure may mask the signs of shock

It is easy to underestimate the extent of blood loss at the time of admission, and in the seriously injured patient it is important to repeat the haemoglobin and haematocrit measurements after volume replacement has been completed. Once haemodilution has taken place the haemoglobin may fall dramatically.

While a degree of haemodilution may be beneficial to cerebral perfusion by reducing viscosity this process, if continued, may lead to levels of circulating haemoglobin insufficient to maintain tissue oxygenation. Therefore, blood losses should be replaced with the aim of maintaining a haemoglobin level of at least 10 g/100 ml and a haematocrit of 30–35%.

Obstruction of cerebral venous return

Obstruction of the venous outflow from the head causes elevation of the intracranial pressure and neurological deterioration. This can be caused by tilting the patient 'head-down' for countertraction or for the insertion of central venous lines. The same effect can be caused by a tight cervical collar in the unconscious patient, and these should be removed as soon as the integrity of the cervical spine is established. This is especially important in the patient who has been paralyzed for ventilation and in whom the neurological deterioration caused by the collar is not evident without an intracranial pressure monitor.

Similar increases in intracranial pressure due to cerebral venous obstruction will result from attempts to intubate the unconscious patient who is capable of resisting. Unless the patient is so deeply unconscious that intubation can be carried out without any difficulty and without provoking gagging and coughing it is necessary to induce anaesthesia (see p. 133).

Epileptic fits

Post-traumatic fits can complicate both severe head injuries and minor head injuries alike. Following the fit there is often a period of reduced consciousness, and if the patient is carefully observed it will become evident that the conscious level is improving. The occurrence of a fit is associated with a small increase in the incidence of intracranial haematoma; but there are always other indications that the patient is developing an intracranial mass. It is not to the advantage of a patient who has just had a fit to be promptly transferred by ambulance to a neurosurgical centre, on the assumption that the event heralds a developing intracranial haematoma. The main risk to the patient is that of respiratory embarrassment in the course of a further fit, and this is difficult to manage in a speeding ambulance.

In the event of a fit the main requirement is to guard the patient's airway. Most fits are self-limiting; but status epilepticus and frequent recurrent fits cause anoxic injury to the brain, and must be controlled. If it is clear that the clonic phase of the fit is slowing and the fit is going to cease spontaneously it is unnecessary to make any attempt to arrest it. The drugs used to treat status epilepticus are sedative and respiratory depressant, and their effects complicate subsequent observation of conscious level.

Status epilepticus

If a fit persists for more than 2–3 minutes it should be arrested. The drugs in common use for this purpose are **diazepam** and **chlormethiazole** (See Box 4.2). Diazepam is the most convenient to use, and is

---

Box 4.2   Treatment of status epilepticus in adults

Diazepam	0–10 mg i.v. in 1 mg aliquots (titrate against effect) i.v. infusion 10–40 mg/hour
Chlormethiazole	0.8% solution i.v. infusion 50–100 ml/hour until fits controlled

administered by slow intravenous (i.v.) injection. It should be given in small aliquots, titrating the dose against the response. Chlormethiazole is administered by intravenous infusion. Both drugs are respiratory depressants, and may cause serious respiratory depression or respiratory arrest even in the small doses used in the head-injured patient. They should only be used when facilities are available to ventilate the patient in the event of a respiratory arrest.

A single intravenous injection of diazepam may be sufficient to control status epilepticus. Treatment should continue with one of the anticonvulsant drugs listed in Box 4.3. Recurrent attacks of status epilepticus or frequent recurrent fits must be controlled by an intravenous infusion of either diazepam or chlormethiazole. Respiration must be closely monitored, and assisted ventilation may be required. The sedation caused by this treatment makes clinical monitoring of the patient's neurological condition difficult, and a CT scan should be performed in order to exclude an intracranial haematoma.

> **Sedative drugs may cause respiratory depression in the head-injured patient**

After a single self-limiting fit the patient should be started on a regular anticonvulsant drug (Box 4.3). In the case of the unconscious patient or the patient with multiple injuries, anticonvulsant drugs must be administered parenterally, and this limits the choice of drug to **phenytoin**, **sodium valproate**, and **phenobarbitone**. The first two drugs are the more commonly used, and in terms of their therapeutic value they are equally effective. Sodium valproate should not be used in women of

Box 4.3   Treatment of fits in adults

Phenytoin	250 mg i.v. (slow i.v. injection)
	250 mg i.v. t.d.s. for 24 hours
	100 mg i.v. t.d.s.
	300 mg oral/day when capable
Phenobarbitone	120 mg i.m.
	60 mg i.m. or oral t.d.s.
Sodium valproate	400–800 mg i.v. over 3–5 minutes
	200 mg i.v. or orally t.d.s.
Carbamazepine	200 mg b.d. increasing to 200 mg q.d.s.

child-bearing age. Phenytoin and sodium valproate are administered intravenously by slow injection (over 3–5 minutes). Because phenytoin may cause cardiac arrhythmias and hypotension, blood pressure and ECG monitoring should be used when the drug is administered intravenously. Phenobarbitone should be given intramuscularly. In each case, a loading dose or a series of loading doses are given in order to establish therapeutic blood concentrations, followed by regular maintenance doses orally or parenterally. If the patient is expected to be able to take oral medication within the next 12 hours carbamazepine may be used instead of the drugs mentioned above. Anticonvulsant therapy in children is discussed in Chapter 8.

Intracranial haematoma

Intracranial haematoma is the only cause of neurological deterioration after head injury that requires operative neurosurgical intervention. The clinical features of an expanding intracranial mass are essentially the same whether it is a subdural, an extradural, or an intracerebral haematoma. The physiological effects of rising intracranial pressure are described in Chapter 1. The outcome of treatment is determined by the severity of the primary brain injury and the size and rapidity of onset of the haematoma. (See Box 4.4.)

Extradural haematoma

Extradural haemorrhage arises from meningeal blood vessels—commonly the middle meningeal vessels—and is the result of a skull injury. Approximately 90% of adult patients with extradural haematoma have demonstrable skull fractures on X-ray. The recognition of a skull fracture, then, is most important in anticipating deterioration due to extradural haematoma. However, in children there is a lower incidence of

Box 4.4   Clinical features of intracranial haematoma

- Headache, vomitting
- Deteriorating conscious level
- Progressive hemiparesis (contralateral)
- Bradycardia, hypertension
- Dilating pupil (ipsilateral)
- Irregular respiration

radiologically recognized skull fracture in association with extradural haematoma (60–70%).

The commonest site for extradural haematomas is in the temporal region, where the skull is thin and the middle meningeal vessels are vulnerable; but haematomas occur at other sites, usually determined by the site of the fracture. The haematoma caused by extradural haemorrhage strips the dura from the inner table of the skull as it increase in volume, and compresses the underlying brain. The effects of the haematoma are due to rising intracranial pressure and localized distortion of the brain.

Since this condition is so often associated with a relatively minor primary injury it is a particular tragedy if it is not recognized and treated.

Symptoms

The primary brain injury may have been minor, and, on occasion, the patient may not have been unconscious at all. In either event, there is often a 'lucid interval' in which the patient may recover consciousness or remain conscious for a number of hours. This period is succeeded by increasing headache, vomiting, and deteriorating consciousness. Focal neurological deficits such as limb weakness or dysphasia may be recognized by the patient or by those in attendance. On some occasions, severe persistent headache alone, without altered consciousness or focal deficit, may be the mode of presentation. Extradural haemorrhage does, of course, also occur in the context of the severe primary injury, in which case it causes further deterioration in the already unconscious patient.

Examination

Associated with the skull fracture there may be a scalp injury. Subgaleal bleeding may give rise to a 'boggy' scalp haematoma. Consciousness may be depressed on the Glasgow Coma Scale; but some patients present with headache and focal neurological signs alone. There may be a contralateral limb weakness or evidence of dysphasia. As the haematoma develops the rising intracranial pressure is accompanied by bradycardia and hypertension, and increasing irregularity of respiration. Eventually, the volume of the haematoma causes herniation of the ipsilateral temporal lobe through the tentorial hiatus, where it impinges on the oculomotor (third cranial) nerve. At this critical stage the ipsilateral pupil becomes dilated, and then ceases to react to light (Fig. 4.1).

Any further increase in the volume of the haematoma will result in dilatation of the contralateral pupil, and unless treatment is instituted immediately, there is little likelihood of recovery.

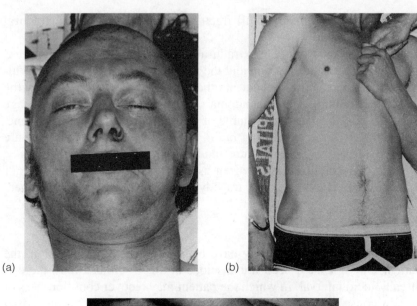

(a)   (b)

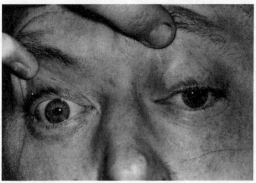

(c)

Fig. 4.1   (a) Right-sided facial weakness in a patient with a left extradural haematoma.
(b) Right limb weakness in a patient with a left extradual haematoma. The right limbs fail
to move in response to a painful stimulus. (c) Dilated left pupil in a patient with a left
extradural haematoma.

Extradural haematomas in the posterior fossa cause rapid deterioration in consciousness and respiratory depression. Tachycardia and
hypotension may be seen, in contrast to the findings in supratentorial
haematomas.

Diagnosis

Neurological deterioration in the presence of a skull fracture is suggestive of an extradural haematoma. The site of the scalp injury and the

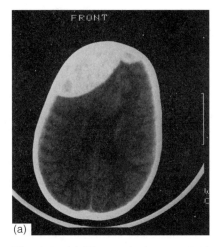 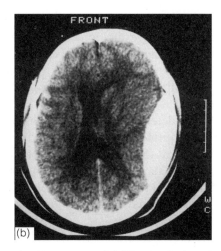

Fig. 4.2   (a) CT scan of a fronto-parietal extradural haematoma; (b) CT scan of a frontal extradural haematoma.

lateralization of the neurological signs indicate whether the lesion is on the left or the right. The haematoma is usually related to the site of the fracture. An extradural haematoma has a characteristic CT scan appearance (Fig. 4.2); but when scanning facilities are not available it may be necessary to proceed to surgery on the basis of the clinical signs and the skull X-ray.

Treatment

The definitive treatment of extradural haematoma requires a craniotomy, in order to remove the haematoma and control bleeding. It is desirable, and possible in most parts of Britain, that this should be done in a neurosurgical unit. Where distance or weather make transfer impossible, the general surgeon may have to be prepared to operate in the base hospital. If the patient's condition is deteriorating rapidly, or if the patient must be transferred to a distant hospital, measures must be taken to prevent further deterioration in transit.

A temporary reduction in intracranial pressure can be achieved by intravenous administration of diuretic agents. Use either **mannitol** or **frusemide**. Mannitol is given as a rapid intravenous infusion, 0.5 g being given per kg body weight. This amounts to 150–200 ml of a 20% solution in an average adult, and it should be infused over 5 minutes. Frusemide is given as an intravenous bolus of 40 mg in an adult or 1 mg/kg body weight in a child. The ensuing diuresis will improve or at least maintain the patient's condition, but only for 1–2 hours; and this treatment may have to be repeated if there is further deterioration before definitive investigations or treatment have been completed. During this time, arrangements must be made as rapidly as possible to ensure that surgical treatment follows. **Diuretics should not be given to hypovolaemic patients**, since they will cause a further reduction in blood volume.

The deteriorating patient with an intracranial haematoma can ill afford any respiratory interruption, and should be anaesthetized, paralysed, and ventilated (See Box 4.5). Hyperventilation will also reduce intracranial pressure (see p. 12). This is an essential measure if the patient is to be transferred to a distant hospital.

Three units of blood should be cross-matched and available in the operating theatre.

A decision must then be made as to whether there is time to permit a CT scan. If not, the surgeon must decide on the site of the haematoma with the aid of the clinical signs and the skull X-ray. It should be remembered that a significant number of extradural haematomas are not found at the classical temporal site, but may be frontal or in the posterior fossa. The haematoma is found **on the same side as the dilated pupil** and on the **opposite** side to the hemiparesis. It is usually located **at the site of the skull fracture**.

An extradural haematoma is a solid clot covering a large area of the surface of the dura, and **cannot be treated through a burr hole**. The ideal surgical procedure is a craniotomy: but, where the surgeon's experience does not permit this, a burr hole can be extended to form a craniectomy by removing bone (see Chapter 9). This will be sufficient to save the patient's life; but the resulting skull defect will make further surgery necessary at a later date.

Box 4.5   Management of deteriorating patient with suspected intracranial haematoma

- Ensure that basic resuscitation is complete
- 20% mannitol i.v. bolus 0.5 g/kg body weight
- Anaesthetize and ventilate
- Maintain paralysis and sedation
- Transfer if necessary
- Cross-match blood 3 units
- CT scan (if time permits)
- Craniotomy (craniectomy if craniotomy impossible)

The problems for the occasional surgeon operating outside a neurosurgical unit are that, first, the site of the lesion may be misjudged; and second, the lesion may not prove to be the expected extradural haematoma, but an acute subdural or intracerebral haematoma. Furthermore, the main surgical challenge is not the removal of the clot, but the arrest of the subsequent bleeding, which can be extremely difficult for the uninitiated surgeon.

Operative surgical technique is discussed in Chapter 9.

Subdural haematoma

Subdural haematoma may be **acute** or **subacute**. The **acute subdural haematoma** is usually associated with a severe primary brain injury, causing further deterioration in the patient's already impaired conscious level and vital signs. The outcome will be determined substantially by the severity of the primary injury.

The **subacute subdural haematoma** develops over a period of days, and is due to haemorrhage from a bridging vein between the brain and the dura, often after relatively trivial trauma. In many instances this phenomenon is made possible by a degree of pre-existing cerebral atrophy. Thus it is commonly seen in alcoholics and the elderly. In the case of the former, alcoholic liver disease contributes the additional factor of impaired blood coagulation.

The clinical course of events is similar to that described for extradural haemorrhage, particularly in the case of the subacute haematoma which may present after a lucid interval. Similar focal neurological signs are seen, associated with bradycardia and hypertension. The finding of a skull fracture is less frequently associated with subdural haematoma.

Diagnosis

The clinical diagnosis of a subdural haematoma (as distinct from an extradural or intracerebral haematoma) cannot be made with any confidence. Its clinical localization is made according to the focal neurological signs (hemiparesis, dilated pupil); but it is impossible to predict on clinical grounds whether the lesion is frontal or parieto-occipital. Acute subdural haematoma has a characteristic CT scan appearance, and the scan allows the surgeon to determine the extent of the haematoma and to plan the surgical approach accordingly (see Fig. 4.3).

In the case of the alcoholic patient with a subacute haematoma it is wise to carry out clotting studies (prothrombin time, INR) and administer vitamin K, 5 mg by slow intravenous injection preoperatively.

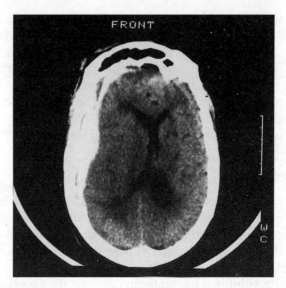

Fig. 4.3   CT scan of an acute subdural haematoma with midline shift.

Treatment

While referral to a neurosurgical unit is being arranged the deteriorating patient can be stabilized by the use of intravenous mannitol 20% and ventilation on the lines described for extradural haematoma.

Subdural haematoma is treated by craniotomy, and since the site of origin of the haemorrhage cannot be determined preoperatively, a large craniotomy is required. If it is clear that the primary injury has been very severe and the patient presents with a very poor level of consciousness and non-reacting pupils, removal of the haematoma is unlikely to be followed by a useful recovery, and surgery is not indicated. Even in the case of the subacute haematoma, results can be disappointing, because the pre-existing cerebral atrophy diminishes the brain's capacity for recovery.

Intracerebral haematoma

Traumatic intracerebral haematoma is, more strictly speaking, an area of haemorrhagic contusion caused by a closed-head injury, and often by the contre-coup mechanism. A common example is that of the patient who falls backwards and strikes the occiput. The frontal lobes are contused as they rebound off the frontal bone, and this may be followed by increasing swelling of the contused brain, leading to progressive neurological deterioration.

The patient usually feels ill with headache, focal neurological deficit, or altered consciousness from the time of the injury, and deteriorates over the course of days. The gradual deterioration may be missed if not carefully observed, until a critical point is reached, when the patient declines rapidly.

Diagnosis

As in the case of the subdural haematoma the nature and site of the lesion cannot be predicted clinically with confidence, and the diagnosis is made by CT scan.

These patients illustrate the dangers in operating on head-injured patients outside a neurosurgical unit without the aid of a scan. The fracture is remote from the haematoma, and the lesion is difficult to localize clinically. The inexperienced surgeon may operate at the wrong site, expecting to find an extradural haematoma at the site of the fracture.

Treatment

These patients require careful observation, preferably with intracranial pressure monitoring. Since the lesion consists of contused brain, some of which may be viable, a conservative approach is followed unless the patient is clearly deteriorating. Swelling of the contused lobe may cause deterioration in the succeeding days, and this may take the form of a gradual deterioration in conscious level, hypertension and bradycardia, and increasing focal neurological deficit. On the other hand, there may be a rapid deterioration, particularly if there is an episode of respiratory impairment or an epileptic fit. It may then be necessary to carry out a craniotomy in order to evacuate the haematoma or to resect the injured lobe.

These patients must be observed in a neurosurgical unit, so that prompt treatment can be instituted.

Fluid balance

Overhydration and hyponatraemia may cause a deterioration in conscious level in the head-injured patient. Part of the early metabolic response to trauma is to retain water. The head-injured patient will often be breathing humidified oxygen, and insensible fluid loss from respiration is largely abolished. **In the absence of other fluid losses no more than 1500 cc of fluid will be required each day in adults**. While the patient is incapable of taking oral fluids daily fluid requirements should be supplied intravenously using a dextrose/saline combination.

After 3–4 days fluids may be given by nasogastric tube until the patient is capable of drinking. The head-injured patient is sensitive to water overload, and over the course of 4 or 5 days of excessive fluids there may be a deterioration in conscious level. The diagnosis is confirmed by the finding of a low serum sodium. Hyponatraemia with a serum sodium of less than 130 mEq/litre may also cause epileptic fits.

It is sufficient simply to stop all fluids until the excess water has been excreted, following which there may be a gradual but gratifying improvement in the patient's neurological condition. Do not give hypertonic saline. This simply exacerbates the problem of fluid overload.

Polyuria may occur for one of two reasons. The patient who is a known or latent diabetic may become hyperglycaemic in response to trauma. This is easily recognized if the urine is tested for sugar after admission. Or fractures of the base of the anterior cranial fossa may be complicated by injuries of the pituitary stalk, resulting in **diabetes insipidus**. If this is not recognized the patient may become seriously dehydrated and hypovolaemic. In this condition, a low urine specific gravity and osmolality is associated with a high serum osmolality, a high haematocrit, and a high plasma sodium concentration. Careful fluid balance is important in the early stages of head-injury management.

Drugs

Sedative drugs should be avoided in the early stages after a head injury, while the patient's conscious level remains depressed. This means that opioid analgesics must be used with care (see p. 43). A deterioration in conscious level may be caused by opioid analgesics or by anticonvulsant agents. Establish whether any potentially sedative drugs have been given prior to deterioration.

Sedative drugs may cause respiratory depression in the head-injured patient

---

A not infrequent culprit is diazepam, administered during an epileptic fit, or, sometimes, even after a fit. The patient then fails to regain the former level of consciousness, and the problem may be compounded by respiratory depression, which, in turn causes further cerebral depression. **Diazepam and related drugs should not be administered to head-injured patients**. The only **exception to this rule** is in the event of status epilepticus, when intravenous diazepam is justified, provided that facilities are immediately available to intubate and ventilate the patient. **Flumazenil** is a specific antidote to benzodiazepines, and may be used if a deterioration in consciousness or respiration is thought to be due to diazepam or related drugs.

Sedative drugs are sometimes given to the head-injured patient who has become restless and uncooperative, having been drowsy and withdrawn initially. This turn of events signals a deterioration, not an improvement, in conscious level, and should raise the question of a developing intracranial haematoma. In these circumstances, sedation is potentially disastrous.

One of the cardinal reasons for admission of the head-injured patient to hospital is to protect the patient from further injury that may otherwise result from avoidable or treatable factors. This is made possible by monitoring conscious level and vital signs. The present chapter has outlined the possible causes of neurological deterioration; and it should be evident that in many instances systemic factors are responsible. Since these complications may require early treatment, it is important that precipitate transfer to a specialist unit should not replace adequate resuscitation.

Further reading

Jennett, B. and Carlin, J. (1978). Preventable mortality and morbidity after head injury. *Injury*, **10**, 31–9.

Jennett, B. and Lindsay, K. W. (1994). *Introduction to neurosurgery*, Heinemann Medical, London.

Jennett, B. and Teasdale, G. (1981). *Management of head injuries*, (Contemporary Neurology Series). F. A. Davis, Philadelphia.

5 Radiology

Chapter contents

Key points in radiology

1 The main purpose of the skull X-ray in cases of trauma is to recognize a fracture and to establish whether or not it is a depressed fracture.
2 A linear fracture is seen as a hard black line, distinct from the normal marks, or as a widening of a suture line, particularly in children. A fracture, unlike vascular markings, may radiate in several directions from a central focus.
3 'Face-on', a depressed fracture is seen as a series of lines radiating from a central focus, or as a circular marking. Viewed tangentially, it is seen as a depression in the contour of the skull.
4 The extradural haematoma appears on a computerized tomography (CT) scan as a lens-shaped lesion that is convex inwardly.
5 The acute subdural haematoma appears on a CT scan as a layer of blood conforming to the surface of the cortex (i.e. concave inwardly).
6 The intracerebral haematoma appears on a CT scan as a patchy area of high density, with compression or shift of the ventricles, and clearly within the substance of the brain.
7 X-rays of the cervical spine should include lateral, antero-posterior, and in the conscious patient, open mouth views showing the odontoid process. The lateral view must include the C7-T1 junction, for which the patient's shoulders must be pulled down during X-ray.
8 The commonest sites for cervical spine injuries are the C1/C2 region and the lower cervical spine (C5-C7), which should be examined on X-rays with particular attention.
9 A haematoma in the paraspinal tissues is seen on the lateral projection as an increase in the pre-spinal soft tissue shadow (greater than 10 mm at the C1/C2 level, and 20 mm at the C5/C6 level in the adult).

The interpretation of skull X-rays often devolves to relatively junior doctors in the A&E department, often at hours when experienced colleagues are not always available. The finding of a skull fracture is important in its own right, in view of the possible complications of the skull injury. It is also important evidence that the patient has had a head injury when no history of trauma is available—for example, when a patient is admitted in an unconscious state of unknown aetiology.

Meningitis, subarachnoid haemorrhage, and epileptic fits may each be due to head trauma and, where no reliable history is available, skull X-rays are required in case the patient is presenting with one of these complications of head injury.

Box 5.1 · Indications for skull X-ray

- History of unconsciousness
- Scalp bruising, haematoma, laceration
- Neurological deficit
- Impaired conscious level
- CSF rhinorrhoea, otorrhoea
- Headache, vomitting
- Unconscious, ? head injury

The head injury may be accompanied by injuries of the cervical spine, and a series of cervical spine X-rays should be obtained in any conscious patient with neck pain and in all patients with altered consciousness. (See Box 5.1.)

Indications for skull X-rays

Skull X-rays are not indicated in all of the very large number of patients attending hospitals each year with head injuries. Undoubtedly, a very large number of normal skull X-rays are carried out every year, and of those that are found to have a skull fracture a small minority develop complications. The complications of the skull injury, however, are both lethal and either treatable or preventable, and expenditure on radiology has to be viewed in this light. Various attempts have been made to rationalize the indications for skull X-rays; but, of course, guidelines are only guidelines, and the attending doctor must judge whether the skull is likely to have been injured according to the nature and severity of the injury.

The normal skull X-ray

In order to recognize abnormalities on the skull X-ray it is necessary to be familiar with the normal radiological anatomy of the skull in each of the conventional projections. When skull X-rays are requested, three views should be provided—an antero-posterior, a lateral, and a Townes projection (see below). On each of these there are certain features which are constant in position, and others that are normal findings, but of variable position and appearance.

Where a depressed fracture is suspected, a tangential view of the area should be taken, so that the suspect area is placed on the 'skyline' of the skull.

The normal markings seen on the skull vault are the **diploic veins** of the skull, the **meningeal vessels**, and the **suture lines**. The diploic veins are inconstant in position, and are seen as broad, soft markings. The **middle meningeal vessels** are constant in position, and more clearly demarcated. They can usually be seen to divide into anterior and posterior branches. Suture lines are characteristically 'saw-toothed' in appearance, and constant in position.

The antero-posterior skull X-ray

The normal antero-posterior (AP) skull X-ray (Fig. 5.1) shows the orbital margins, the frontal and ethmoid sinuses, the sagittal suture, and the lambdoid sutures, as well as the diploic veins.

The pineal gland may be seen as a calcified structure just above the eyebrows in the midline.

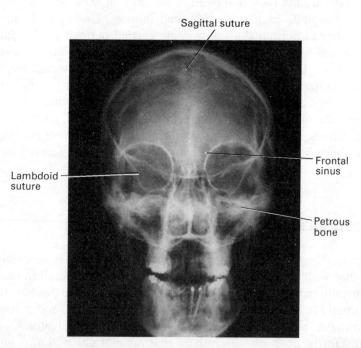

Fig. 5.1   Normal skull X-ray: antero-posterior view.

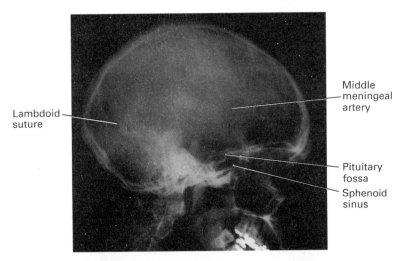

Lambdoid suture

Middle meningeal artery

Pituitary fossa

Sphenoid sinus

Fig. 5.2 Normal skull X-ray: lateral view.

The lateral skull X-ray

The normal lateral skull X-ray (Fig. 5.2) shows the frontal sinuses and the sphenoid sinus. The other 'fixed' features are the coronal suture and the middle meningeal artery, which divides into an anterior and a posterior branch. The other normal features are the diploic veins of the skull, which are randomly distributed, and are seen as soft shadows. The pineal gland is often calcified, and is seen just above the pinna of the ear. If it is clearly visible on this view it may also be identifiable on the AP or Townes views, where it is more difficult to recognize.

The Townes view

This fronto-occipital projection shows the occipital bone. Note the normal features, which include the lambdoid sutures and the foramen magnum. The pineal gland may be visible as a midline calcified structure (Fig. 5.3).

The abnormal skull X-ray (skull fractures)

The main purpose of the skull X-ray in cases of trauma is to recognize a fracture and to establish whether it is a depressed fracture. Of occasional value is the demonstration of a shift of midline structures by showing a lateral displacement of a calcified pineal gland.

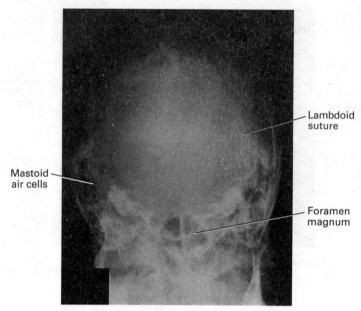

Fig. 5.3   Normal skull X-ray: Townes view.

A linear fracture is seen as a hard black line, distinct from the normal markings (Fig. 5.4). Alternatively, there may be widening of a suture line, particularly in children. A fracture, unlike vascular markings, may radiate in several directions from a central focus. Skull fractures remain radiologically evident for many years after injury, and it can be impossible to determine whether a fracture is recent or old unless previous X-rays are available for comparison.

'Face-on', a depressed fracture is seen as a series of lines radiating from a central focus, or as a circular marking. Viewed tangentially, it is seen as a depression in the contour of the skull. The inner table of the skull may be depressed to a greater extent than the outer, and spicules of bone can be seen angled inwards (Fig. 5.5).

Fractures of the skull base are often very difficult to detect on the standard projections above, and are recognized by indirect evidence. Since these fractures often involve the air sinuses they may result in blood or cerebrospinal fluid (CSF) occupying the sinuses. Typically, the sphenoid sinus is seen to contain fluid, which appears as an air–fluid level. Since the lateral skull view is taken with the patient lying horizontally and brow-up, the fluid level is best recognized by viewing the X-ray with the film in this orientation (Fig. 5.6).

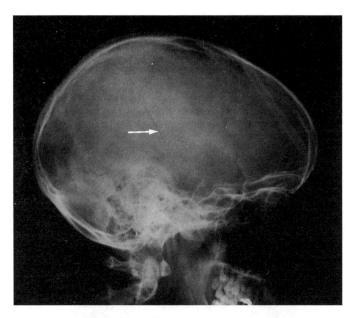

Fig. 5.4 Abnormal skull X-ray: linear fracture.

In basal skull fractures involving the sinuses and other compound injuries, penetration of the dura allows escape of CSF and entry of air into the cranial cavity. This is seen as black 'bubbles' within the skull. In the case of an anterior fossa fracture with CSF rhinorrhoea, a large quantity of air may occupy the anterior fossa as an aerocele (Fig. 5.7).

The CT scan

The indications for a CT scan are described in Chapter 3 (p. 42). In many instances it is necessary to transport the patient to another hospital if a scan is required. It is vital to ensure that the patient has been resuscitated adequately before being moved. Close observation and resuscitation facilities remain necessary during the scan. It is impossible to scan a moving patient, and in the case of the very restless patient a decision has to be taken as to whether to carry out the scan under general anaesthetic or to adopt a close watching policy and proceed to the scan if the patient's conscious level deteriorates or any focal neurological signs develop. The latter course is more safely conducted in a neurosurgical unit. Sedation with diazepam or other similar agents should not be used, because of the serious danger of inducing respiratory depression.

Depressed fracture

(a)

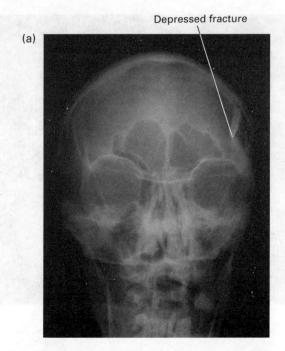

(b)

Depressed fracture

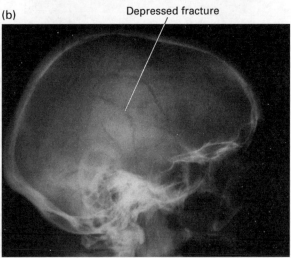

Fig. 5.5   Abnormal skull X-ray: depressed fracture. (a) Frontal view; (b) lateral view.

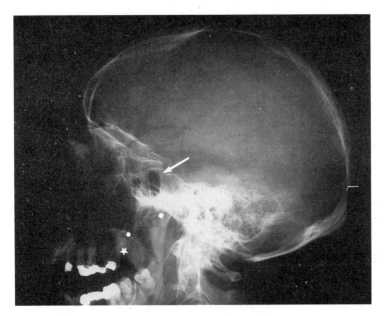

Fig. 5.6   Abnormal skull X-ray: air-fluid level in a sinus.

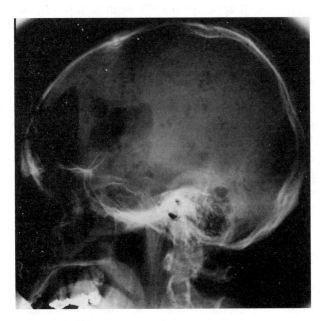

Fig. 5.7   Abnormal skull X-ray: an aerocele.

Do not sedate the restless patient for a CT scan

Figs. 4.2–4.4 show examples of CT abnormalities.

Extradural haematoma

Note that the extradural haematoma appears on a CT scan as a lens-shaped lesion that is convex inwardly. The associated skull fracture may be evident on the scan. The degree of ventricular shift gives an indication of the extent of the mass effect of the haematoma.

Subdural haematoma

The acute subdural haematoma appears on a CT scan as a layer of blood conforming to the surface of the cortex (i.e. concave inwardly).

Intracerebral haematoma/contusion

The intracerebral haematoma following trauma is usually a haemorrhagic contusion in which brain and blood are mixed to varying degrees. It is rarely a discrete clot. It appears on a CT scan as a patchy area of high density, with compression or shift of the ventricles, and is clearly within the substance of the brain.

Diffuse brain injury

Diffuse brain injury without extracerebral or intracerebral haematoma may present with CT evidence of brain swelling alone. The ventricles appear smaller than would be expected, taking into consideration the age of the patient. The basal cisterns may be effaced or absent. Small areas of haemorrhage may be seen scattered throughout the brain, but particularly in the corpus callosum. Severe diffuse brain injury may occur without any unequivocal abnormality on the CT scan.

X-rays of the cervical spine

The initial X-rays of the cervical spine must be obtained without moving the patient from the resuscitation trolley. Routine examination of the cervical spine should include a lateral view, an antero-posterior view, and in the conscious patient, an open mouth view, to show the odontoid process. The lateral view must include the junction of C7 and T1. To achieve this the patient's shoulders must be pulled down by applying traction to the arms while the X-ray is taken. If this fails to demonstrate the lower cervical spine a 'swimmer's view' should be obtained by raising one of the arms above the head while the other is held downwards and behind the patient's back. These X-rays will show deformity of the spine, fractures of the vertebral bodies, and loss of normal alignment, and are sufficient for the early stages of management. Further views may be required later if the patient complains of symptoms such as neck pain or paraesthesia in the limbs.

The commonest sites for cervical spine injuries are the C1/C2 region and the lower cervical spine (C5–C7). Particular attention should be paid to those areas when the X-rays are examined.

Interpretation

The X-rays must be examined, first, for evidence of a spinal injury, and, second, for evidence of instability. Examine each of the vertebral bodies in turn in the AP and lateral projections, noting obvious fractures or any alteration of the normal oblong outline (Fig. 5.8). Small triangular

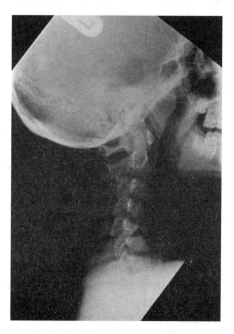

Fig. 5.8 Abnormal cervical spine X-ray: a vertebral fracture.

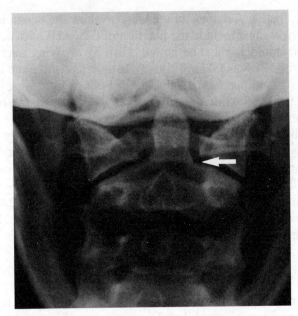

Fig. 5.9   Open-mouth X-ray: a fracture of the odontoid process.

fragments may be avulsed from the anterior borders of the vertebral body in potentially unstable injuries without loss of alignment. In the lateral projection, examine the spinous processes for fractures. Examine the open-mouth view for evidence of fractures of the odontoid process (Fig. 5.9).

Inspect the lateral and AP views for loss of alignment. In the lateral projection the anterior and posterior surfaces of the vertebrae form a smooth anteriorly curving line. An abrupt loss of continuity in these lines indicates a subluxation or dislocation of the spine at this level (Fig. 5.10).

The disc spaces should also be examined. Widening of the disc space either anteriorly or posteriorly indicates disruption of the anterior or posterior longitudinal ligaments, and potential instability. Narrowing of the disc space may occur if there has been traumatic rupture of the disc.

At the level of the injury there may be a haematoma in the paraspinal tissues. This is seen on the lateral projection as an increase in the pre-spinal soft tissue shadow. At the C1/C2 level, the soft tissue shadow should not exceed 10 mm in the adult, and at the C5/C6 level it should be less than 20 mm. An increase in the soft tissue shadow may be seen in the absence of any obvious fracture or loss of alignment (Fig. 5.11).

If, after the standard views, there remains suspicion of a spinal injury further X-rays may be indicated. Oblique 45° views show the pedicles

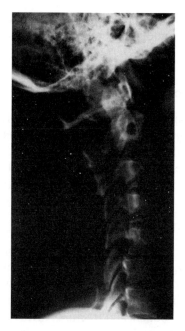

Fig. 5.10   Abnormal cervical spine X-ray: a loss of alignment in the spine.

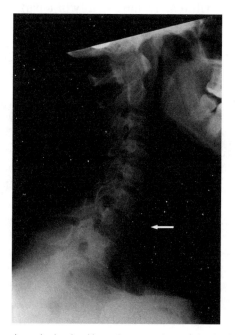

Fig. 5.11   Abnormal cervical spine X-ray: increased pre-spinal soft tissue shadow.

and facet joints, which are less readily defined on the AP and lateral projections. Conventional tomography and views in flexion and extension may be indicated.

CT scan of the cervical spine

Computerized tomography (CT) has made an important contribution to the evaluation of the injured cervical spine. A number of fractures which cannot be demonstrated by conventional radiography are shown by CT scanning. Furthermore, CT is capable of demonstrating in detail the configuration of the fracture and its potential instability (Fig. 5.12).

Radiological assessment of stability

The stability of a cervical spine injury depends on the site and configuration of fractures, the presence of ligamentous injuries, and the mechanism of the injury. Certain fractures must always be regarded as unstable. Fractures of the odontoid process belong to this category. Burst fractures of the vertebral bodies and fractures involving the facet joints or lateral masses of other vertebrae should be assumed to be unstable. Evidence of disruption of the anterior or posterior spinal ligaments or the interspinous ligaments with or without loss of alignment indicate potential instability. Ultimately, the stability of a particular fracture may have to be tested by carefully controlled flexion and extension views; but these should not be taken in the A&E department. The patient should be admitted under the care of a neurosurgeon or orthopaedic surgeon, and

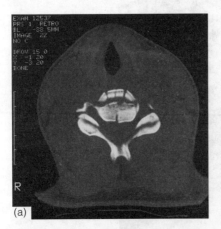 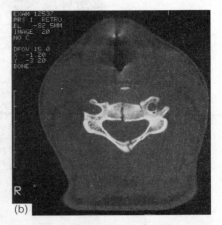

Fig. 5.12   CT scan of a cervical spine fracture. (a) Comminuted fracture of vertebral body; (b) fracture of vertebral body and lamina.

flexion/extension views should be taken only after consultation with an experienced radiologist.

Further reading

Anon. (1984). Guidelines for initial management after head injury in adults: suggestions from a group of neurosurgeons. *British Medical Journal*, **288**, 983–5.

Anon. (1987). Skull X-ray examinations after head trauma: recommendations by a multidisciplinary panel and validation study. *New England Journal of Medicine*, **316**, 84–91.

Meyer, P. R. (1989). *Surgery of spine trauma*, (chapter X). complete reference Churchill Livingstone, New York.

Mirvis, S. and Young, J. (1992). *Imaging in trauma and critical care*. Williams and Wilkins, Baltimore.

Raby, N., Berman, L., and de Lacy, G. (1995). *Accident and emergency radiology: a survival guide*. W.B. Saunders Co Ltd, New York.

Tyson, G. W. (1987). *Head injury management for providers of emergency care*, pp. 121–68. Williams & Wilkins, Baltimore.

6 *Scalp and skull injuries*

Chapter contents

Key points in scalp and skull injuries

1   Bruising of the mastoid processes behind the ears is evidence of a fracture of the petrous bone, which in turn indicates the patient may be at risk of meningitis from a fracture communicating with the middle ear cavity.
2   Extracranial haematomas are recognized as characteristically 'boggy' swellings in the scalp overlying the fracture.
3   Unless a careful clinical examination of the scalp (which is also important for medico-legal reasons) is carried out, serious penetrating injuries may easily be missed if the wound is small. Failure to recognize the possibility that a small scalp injury may be deeply penetrating may expose the patient to the risk of meningitis or cerebral abscess.
4   The scalp of a child with a subgaleal haematoma is tense and fluctuant, and the child may be distressed, restless, and febrile. The haematoma can be aspirated with a syringe and a large-bore needle, but only in an operating theatre with full aseptic precautions—not as an outpatient procedure.
5   Where scalp lacerations involve skin loss or are cosmetically important wounds should be closed by a plastic surgeon, as wound closure without tension can become very difficult. Heavy blood loss is to be expected.
6   'Scalping' injuries involve serious blood loss, and there is a danger the skin flap may become ischaemic.
7   Skull base fractures in the anterior fossa are recognized clinically by the presence of periorbital haematomas or subconjunctival haemorrhages, and by evidence of cerebrospinal fluid (CSF) rhinorrhoea. They may be complicated by meningitis: therefore the patient should be treated with prophylactic antibiotics for one week from the time of injury or the cessation of CSF rhinorrhoea or otorrhoea.
8   Patients with scalp lacerations and underlying fractures should also be given prophylactic antibiotics.
9   Patients presenting with headache, fever, and focal neurological signs some weeks or months after a penetrating head injury should excite a suspicion of a subdural empyema. Meningism may be present, but the presence of focal signs should deter lumbar puncture until empyema has been excluded—the raised intracranial pressure (ICP) of empyema could render lumbar puncture lethal. Patients should be referred to a neurosurgeon if this diagnosis is suspected.

Scalp injuries

Significance of scalp injuries

The scalp injury both draws attention to the fact that the patient has had a head injury and may itself be of serious significance. Failure to recognize that the patient has had a head injury may mean that, in the event of deterioration, the possibility of intracranial haemorrhage is not considered.

The unconscious patient presenting in the A&E department may have had a head injury, and this is sometimes not clear from the history. A careful search of the scalp is an essential part of the examination in order to identify the signs of trauma. These may be relatively slight and obscured by hair. Gently palpate the whole scalp in order to recognize scalp haematomas, and part the hair to look for lacerations or contusions. Always look behind the ears for bruising of the mastoid processes, which is evidence of a fracture of the petrous bone; and this in turn indicates that the patient may be at risk of meningitis from a fracture communicating with the middle ear cavity.

Skull fractures are associated with both extracranial and intracranial haemorrhage. Extracranial haematomas are recognized as characteristically **'boggy' swellings** in the scalp overlying the fracture. This may be easier for the novice to recognize than the radiological appearance of the fracture.

Scalp injuries draw attention to possible skull injuries

The scalp injury may be of some medico-legal significance, and it is important to record both the number of injuries and their appearance. Unless a careful clinical examination of the scalp is carried out, serious penetrating injuries may easily be missed if the external wound is small. The patient, whose X-ray is shown in Fig. 6.1, was not recognized to have a penetrating head injury until his skull was X-rayed.

Failure to recognize the possibility that a small scalp injury may be deeply penetrating may expose the patient to the risk of meningitis or cerebral abscess.

In children, a scalp injury may be complicated by bleeding in the subgaleal layer of the scalp. The scalp of the patient with a **subgaleal haematoma** is tense and fluctuant. (See also Fig. 6.2) The condition can be very painful, and the child may be distressed, restless, and febrile. If

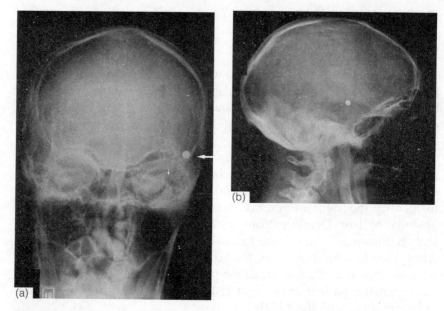

Fig. 6.1   Skull X-ray showing bullet. (a) Antero-posterior view; (b) lateral view.

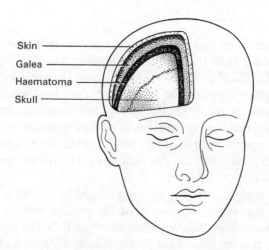

Fig. 6.2   Diagram of scalp layers and subgaleal haematoma.

this condition causes severe symptoms the haematoma should be aspirated with a syringe and a large-bore needle; but great caution should be exercised, since infection of the subgaleal haematoma is a serious complication. Aspiration should be carried out in an operating theatre with full aseptic precautions, and not as an outpatient procedure.

The younger the child the greater the proportion of the total blood volume that may be thus sequestrated in the scalp; and an infant with a large scalp haematoma may have lost a significant proportion of the circulating blood volume.

Scalp lacerations

The majority of scalp lacerations are simple linear lacerations requiring wound closure under local anaesthetic. More extensive lacerations are more appropriately dealt with under general anaesthesia. Where there are cosmetic considerations or where there is actual skin loss this is best handled by a plastic surgeon, as even a relatively small loss of skin can make wound closure without tension extremely difficult.

The scalp is a very vascular structure, and the blood loss from an extensive laceration can be considerable. The patient may be capable of compensating by vasoconstriction, only to reveal the extent of the blood loss at the induction of anaesthesia, when the blood pressure may drop alarmingly.

The scalp laceration affords an opportunity for the doctor to inspect the skull directly for fractures, and a careful inspection of the wound and palpation with a sterile gloved finger should always be performed to detect any underlying skull injury.

Management of scalp lacerations

For the majority of simple linear scalp lacerations it is sufficient to clean and suture the wound under local anaesthetic: 1% **lignocaine** should be used combined with **adrenaline** 1/200 000.

During inspection and suturing of the wound, blood loss can be controlled by the pressure of an assistant's fingertips along the wound margins (Fig. 6.3). Bleeding will cease after the wound is sutured. It is inefficient and unnecessary to attempt to ligate individual bleeding points.

As with wounds elsewhere, devitalized tissue should be excised. If this is likely to leave a scalp defect that cannot be closed without tension it is quite acceptable to clean and dress the wound and seek plastic surgery advice. Where there is loss of skin it is necessary to be prepared to rotate a scalp flap and cover the donor area with a split skin graft. This will

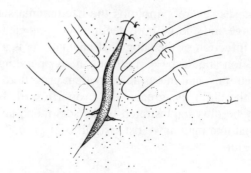

Fig. 6.3   Finger pressure controlling scalp bleeding.

require a general anaesthetic and a surgeon with plastic surgery experience. It is even more important to be sure of sound scalp healing if there
is an underlying fracture.

When it is anticipated that the wound may be difficult to close without
tension it is wise to consider suturing the wound under general anaesthetic, since infiltration with local anaesthetic can further restrict the
mobility of the skin edges.

Before suturing the wound, the scalp should be shaved around the
margins of the lacerations so that it can be adequately cleaned and the
true extent of the injury can be seen.

Most scalp wounds can be closed with a single layer of interrupted
non-absorbable sutures of 2/0 or 3/0 gauge. Sutures are usually removed
after 5 days.

'Scalping' injuries are a rare but serious variety of scalp wound
(Fig. 6.4). Where a large part of the scalp is avulsed there may be serious
blood loss, and there is a danger that the skin flap may be rendered
ischaemic.

Skull injuries

Skull fractures may be closed or compound, or linear or depressed, and
may involve the skull vault or the skull base. The latter may involve the
paranasal or mastoid air sinuses and the cranial nerves as they pass
through the skull base. The fracture may require treatment in its own
right, or may be significant because of its potential complications.

The presence of a skull fracture is among the important indications
for admission to hospital after a head injury, and it is necessary to be
able to recognize both the clinical and the radiological signs.

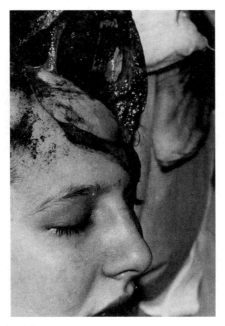

Fig. 6.4 A scalping injury.

Like scalp injuries, skull fractures draw attention to the fact that the patient has had a head injury. A skull X-ray is a necessary investigation in the assessment of the unconscious patient when a reliable history is not available.

Closed fractures

The linear fracture does not require treatment in its own right. Both linear and depressed fractures, however, may be complicated by intracranial haemorrhage. Even in the conscious and orientated patient (i.e. those with Glasgow Coma Scores of 13–14) the presence of a skull fracture is associated with a risk of intracranial haematoma of 1 in 30, and these patients must be admitted to hospital for observation. The significance of the fracture is increased if the patient is not fully conscious. In these circumstances 1 in 4 patients will have some form of intracranial haematoma, and all such patients will require a computerized tomography (CT) scan.

The closed depressed fracture shares the properties of the linear fracture, but may also be disfiguring. This is usually when the fracture is situated outside the hairline in the frontal region.

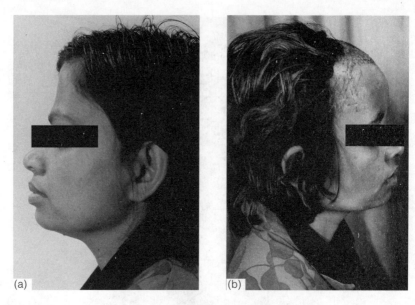

Fig. 6.5   A depressed frontal fracture. (a) Before operation; (b) after operation.

Depressed fractures elsewhere are generally covered by hair (Fig. 6.5), and do not present a cosmetic problem. A disfiguring frontal depressed fracture requires to be elevated on cosmetic grounds; but a closed depressed fracture behind the hairline can usually be left untreated.

Compound skull fractures

Skull fractures may be compound either when there is an overlying scalp wound, in which case the injury may penetrate the dura or brain, or if the fracture involves the air sinuses or the cribriform plate. In either case there is a risk of infective complications.

Skull fractures may be complicated by extradural or other intracranial haematomas

Skull fracture together with altered consciousness indicates a 25% chance of intracranial haematoma

Skull base fractures

Skull base fractures in the anterior fossa are recognized clinically by the presence of periorbital haematomas (Fig. 6.6), or subconjunctival haemorrhages, and by evidence of cerebrospinal fluid (CSF) rhinorrhoea. The nature of the injury should also alert the doctor to the possibility of an anterior fossa fracture. Nasal and facial fractures are associated with damage to the skull base.

Fractures of the petrous bone may involve the middle ear cavity and the mastoid air cells. This may be clinically evident if there is bruising over the mastoid bone or blood, or CSF issuing from the external meatus.

Fractures of the petrous bone may also be accompanied by haemorrhage into the middle ear and disruption of the middle ear apparatus, resulting in haemotympanum and deafness.

The radiological detection of these fractures may be very difficult using standard views. Since these fractures involve the air sinuses, he cribriform plate, or the middle ear and mastoid air cells, they may be complicated by persisting cerebrospinal fluid rhinorrhoea or otorrhoea, and by **meningitis** (see Chapter 12, pp. 174–6).

Skull base fractures may be complicated by meningitis

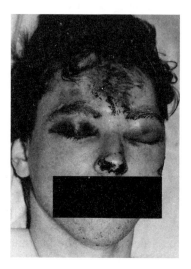

Fig. 6.6 Periorbital haematomas.

Skull base fractures and the risk of meningitis

The main significance of a skull base fracture is that it may be complicated by bacterial meningitis. It was, until recently, common practice to treat patients with skull base fractures with prophylactic antibiotics for an arbitrary period. This practice was based on no good scientific evidence and recent studies have found no justification for it. In some cases, CSF rhinorrhoea is obvious and requires surgical treatment if it does not resolve spontaneously. However, occult CSF leakage can continue over months or years and delayed meningitis is well recognized—sometimes many years after the injury. There can be no rational basis, therefore, for an arbitrary one- or two-week course of antibiotics. Patients with skull base fractures should be observed for signs of meningitis and continuing CSF rhinorrhoea or otorrhoea, and antibiotics introduced only if there is evidence of meningitis.

By far the most common organism involved in post-traumatic meningitis is *Streptococcus pneumoniae* which is a commensal in the nasopharynx. This organism is almost universally sensitive to **benzyl penicillin** which should be given intravenously if meningitis is suspected. A prior lumbar puncture is desirable but this is only permissable when the patient is known not to have an intracranial mass. Meningitis can complicate skull base fractures within hours of the injury.

A variety of commensal organisms are found in the middle ear, including Gram-negative and anaerobic species. Immediate treatment of meningitis arising from a CSF fistula into the middle ear cavity must cover the possibility of infection by a variety of organisms. In the case of proven bacterial meningitis, antibiotic therapy should continue until the cell count in the CSF has returned to normal and, in the case of a demonstrable CSF fluid fistula, until the fistula has been surgically repaired.

Compound linear fractures of the skull vault

It is important, when dealing with a scalp laceration, to establish whether there is an underlying skull fracture. This requires direct inspection and a skull X-ray. In compound linear fractures there is a small risk of meningitis and this can be avoided by attention to cleaning the wound, adequate would excision, and wound closure. Prophylactic antibiotics are not required unless the wound becomes frankly infected, in which case the organism responsible is almost always *Staphylococcus aureus*.

Compound depressed fractures

An innocent-looking laceration may be associated with a depressed fracture of the underlying skull. This should be recognized when the wound is explored or from the X-ray. Evidence of depression of the fracture may not be obvious unless a tangential view of the injured area of the skull is obtained (see Fig. 5.5). Although, on direct inspection, the outer table of the skull may appear to be minimally depressed, the inner table may be much more depressed, with penetration of the underlying structures. These features may be more obvious on the skull X-ray or the CT scan (Fig. 6.7).

Penetrating brain injuries carry the additional risk of **cerebral abscess**, as depressed bone fragments may penetrate the meninges and the brain. Along with fragments of bone, hair, road dirt, and other debris may contaminate the wound. These injuries must be taken very seriously, since the complications are both easily avoided and potentially lethal.

All compound depressed fractures must be surgically explored

An inadequately treated compound head injury may also result in osteomyelitis of the skull and the relatively rare complication of

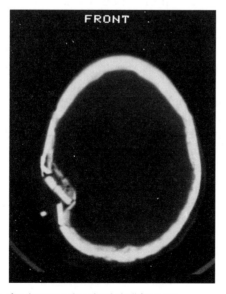

Fig. 6.7 CT scan of a depressed parietal skull fracture.

subdural empyema. The patient usually presents with headache, fever, and focal neurological signs some weeks or even months after a penetrating head injury. Meningism may be present; but the history and the presence of focal signs should deter the doctor from carrying out a lumbar puncture until an empyema has been excluded. This condition causes raised intracranial pressure, which makes lumbar puncture potentially lethal. Subdural empyema can usually be recognized by CT scanning; but the CT appearances may be subtle, and a high index of clinical suspicion is important. If the diagnosis is suspected the patient should be referred to a neurosurgeon.

Some compound head injuries caused by high-velocity impacts or missile injuries may present a spectacular appearance, with exposure or extrusion of brain tissue through the fracture. These injuries are usually associated with more diffuse brain injuries, and it is important that the clinician is not distracted by the grotesque head wound to the detriment of the primary task of resuscitating the patient. The scalp wound should be dressed with cotton swabs and a bandage, and dealt with more definitively once the patient's condition has been stabilized. Urgent neurosurgical attention is therefore not primarily required at this stage, until the patient's resuscitation is complete.

Compound depressed fractures must **always** be explored formally in the operating theatre. In the case of the simple laceration with a shallow depressed fracture it is sufficient to extend the wound and elevate the fracture so that the dura can be inspected for lacerations (see Chapter 9). Care should be exercised in elevating fractures over one of the major venous sinuses; and it is unwise for the inexperienced surgeon to explore a depressed fracture in the midline of the head or over the occiput.

Penetrating brain injuries should be explored, and both debris and contaminated or devitalized tissues should be removed in order to prevent cerebral abscess.

Patients with penetrating head injuries should be treated with prophylactic antibiotics as described above. In the case of compound injuries of the skull vault, the most likely contaminating organism is *Staphy. aureus*, and the choice of antibiotic must be made with this in mind.

Box 6.1   Complications of compound skull injury

- Meningitis
- Cerebral abscess
- Subdural empyema
- Aerocele

Complications of skull fracture

Cerebrospinal fluid leakage

Fractures of the skull base may be complicated by the development of a cerebrospinal fluid (CSF) leak through either the anterior fossa floor or the petrous bone. In the first instance, CSF discharges into the paranasal sinuses or directly into the nose. In the case of petrous bone fractures, the CSF discharges into the middle ear cavity or the mastoid air cells. If the tympanic membrane is intact the fluid then passes down the Eustachian tube to the nasopharynx and presents as CSF rhinorrhoea. Alternatively, it may discharge from the external meatus as CSF otorrhoea. In some patients there is an unrecognized CSF fistula, if the CSF does not appear in the nose or ear and is swallowed instead. This, of course, may persist unrecognized for years and is a cause of delayed meningitis following head injury.

A dilute, watery discharge is reasonably assumed to be CSF but the diagnosis is less certain when the discharge is bloodstained. Epistaxis will generally cease within 24 hours and a persisting bloodstained discharge should be treated as a CSF fistula. There can be uncertainty about the nature of a watery nasal discharge. It used to be taught that CSF can be distinguished from nasal secretions by its glucose content but this is now regarded as unreliable and the accepted laboratory test is now the detection of beta-ferritin in the specimen.

The patient with a CSF fistula should be admitted to hospital. Prophylactic antibiotics should not be given but the staff should be aware of the risk of meningitis. The patient should be advised not to blow the nose since this may cause an **aerocoele** in the anterior fossa (see Fig. 6.8). This collection of air under pressure acts as a mass in the anterior fossa and can cause severe headache, altered consciousness, and meningitis. This phenomenon should be remembered as an occasional cause of acute deterioration in the head-injured patient.

In the majority of patients the CSF fistula will close spontaneously and no surgical treatment is required. Opinions vary as to how long one should wait before resorting to surgical repair of the fistula. There are some surgeons who would advocate active treatment in all cases but most neurosurgeons would delay surgery in the expectation that the fistula will close spontaneously. The fact that there is no obvious rhinorrhoea does not mean that the patient is not still leaking small quantities of CSF and one can attempt to provoke nasal discharge by asking the patient to lie prone across the bed with the head hanging down. In this position, the intracranial pressure will be raised and CSF will tend to appear in the nose if a fistula persists.

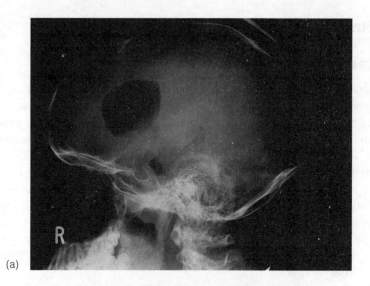

(a)

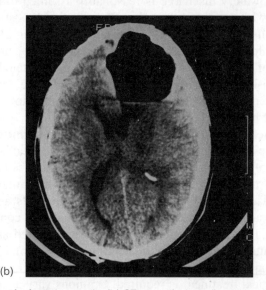

(b)

Fig. 6.8   (a) X-ray of a frontal aerocele; (b) CT scan of a large frontal aerocele.

Cranial nerve injuries

Fractures of the skull base may be complicated by cranial-nerve injuries (Box 6.2). Cranial nerve injuries also occur in the absence of fractures.

Box 6.2 Complications of skull fracture

- Intracranial haematoma
- Cerebrospinal fluid fistula
- Cranial nerve injury
- Cosmetic deformity
- Aerocele

The olfactory nerves are injured in 5–10% of closed head injuries. The impact causes shearing of the olfactory nerves as they pass through the cribriform plate; or the nerve may be injured in fractures of the anterior cranial fossa. The symptoms are usually of little concern to the patient in the immediate period after the injury; but on recovery the loss of the sense of smell can be distressing. Taste is impaired, and the enjoyment of food is spoiled. These impairments may also have implications in certain occupations where the sense of smell or taste is important. They are certainly regarded as a significant consequence of injury in subsequent litigation.

Optic nerve injuries are mercifully uncommon. They tend to occur in severe frontal and facial injuries, such as are seen in road traffic accidents when the front occupants of the car are thrown through the windscreen. The injury may involve the nerve itself or the optic chiasm. The visual fields must be assessed as soon as the patient is able to open the eyes. The light reflex may be absent or reduced; but the consensual reflex operates when the light is shone in the uninjured eye. The 'fixed pupil' in this case should not be confused with that resulting from a third (oculomotor) cranial nerve lesion. The injured optic nerve is capable of recovering with time. Surgical intervention is not helpful.

Diplopia may be due either to injuries of the third, fourth, or sixth cranial nerves, or, more commonly, to bony injuries of the orbit. **The oculomotor (third) cranial nerve** may be injured directly by the impact. The pupil of the affected eye is dilated, and the light reflex is impaired. This is associated with a palsy of the extraocular muscles served by the third nerve, and occasionally with a ptosis. The extraocular palsy is most evident as a weakness of the medial rectus muscle. The patient complains of diplopia on looking to the side of the injured nerve. A dilated pupil also occurs in direct trauma to the eye, in which case there is usually no associated extraocular palsy, and there is evidence of direct trauma to the orbit in the form of bruising or abrasions on the orbital margins, conjunctival injuries, and intraocular blood. The patient with a direct eye injury or an isolated third nerve injury will be conscious and otherwise relatively well. The patient who develops a third nerve palsy as a result of an expanding intracranial mass, on the other hand, is not conscious, and has other signs associated with a severe head injury. The two situations should be readily distinguished.

Injuries of the **fourth (trochlear) nerve** and the **sixth (abducent) nerve** occur in 1–9% of all head injuries. The former causes weakness of the superior oblique muscle and diplopia on downward gaze. The latter affects the lateral rectus muscle, and causes diplopia on gaze to the opposite side. Fortunately, injuries of the third, fourth, and sixth cranial nerves tend to resolve spontaneously. Diplopia is treated in the first instance by providing an eyepatch. If there is persisting diplopia this can be corrected by the provision of prism lenses.

The fifth (trigeminal) nerve is usually injured in fractures of the facial skeleton, resulting in numbness over the cheek.

The facial nerve is injured extracranially in direct blows to the pre-auricular area, and intracranially in fractures of the petrous bone. The facial palsy may be delayed, in which case it is presumed that the progressive facial palsy is attributable to swelling of the nerve within its canal. The extent of the palsy may be limited if the patient is given a short course of corticosteroids. **Prednisolone** 80 mg/day should be prescribed as early as possible after the facial weakness becomes apparent, and continued for 4 to 5 days. The drug should be stopped if there is no response at that stage, or phased out gradually over a longer period if recovery is apparent. This injury is often associated with bruising of the mastoid, and there may be an accompanying injury of the middle ear and CSF otorrhoea.

Middle-ear injuries may result in deafness and bleeding from the external meatus. Inspection with the otoscope will show whether there is a laceration of the external meatus and whether there is a haemotympanum. Again, there is usually no immediate treatment required. A haemotympanum will resolve spontaneously; but persisting deafness may be due to injury of the **acoustic nerve** or the ossicles, and the patient should be referred for the opinion of an ENT surgeon.

Symptoms related to middle-ear and acoustic-nerve injuries are common after head injury, and frequently bring patients back to the Accident Department for advice.

Injuries of the lower cranial nerves occur rarely, and are due to fracture of the occipital bone in the region of the jugular and hypoglossal foramina.

Further reading

Braakman, R. (1972). Depressed skull fracture: data, treatment and follow-up in 225 consecutive cases. *Journal of Neurology, Neurosurgery, and Psychiatry*, **35**, 396–402.

de Louvois, J. *et al.* (1994). Antimicrobial prophylaxis in neurosurgery after head injury. *Lancet*, **334**, 1547–51.

Leech, P. (1974). Cerebrospinal fluid leakage, dural fistulae and meningitis after basal skull fracture. *Injury*, **6**, 141–9.

Tyson, G. W. (1987). *Head injury management for providers of emergency care*, pp. 120–35. Williams & Wilkins, Baltimore.

Vinken, P. J. and Bruyn, G. W. (ed.)(1969). *Handbook of clinical neurology*, vol. 24 (Cranial Nerve Injuries).

Further reading

7 *Cervical spine injuries*

Chapter contents

Key points in cervical spine injury

1 In cases of severe head injury there is a 5–10% incidence of spinal injury.
2 Unconscious head-injured patients should be assumed to have a spinal injury.
3 The cervical spine should be immobilized using a hard collar at the scene of the accident.
4 In-line traction should be applied if the patient is moved.
5 X-rays of the cervical spine should be obtained while resuscitation is carried out.
6 Normal alignment on lateral X-rays does not exclude unstable spinal injury.
7 The neck must be immobilized until spinal injury has been excluded.
8 The lateral cervical spinal X-ray must include the C7/T1 junction.
9 If the patient is immobilized for a prolonged period he/she must be turned regularly to prevent pressure sores.
10 The injured spinal cord is vulnerable to further insults, including compression if there is instability, hypoxia, hypotension, and anaemia.

In victims of trauma, the head and neck should be considered as a single unit. The forces responsible for head injuries also cause injuries of the cervical spine and the two conditions are commonly associated. In one autopsy series of 312 fatal road traffic accidents, 10% had combined head and cervical spine injuries. In unconscious head-injured patients who have been injured in falls or road traffic accidents there is a 5–10% risk of a coexisting cervical spine injury.

Conscious patients are able to give an account of symptoms that draw attention to the possibility of a cervical spine injury.

Head injury is commonly associated with injury of the cervical spine

---

Patients who have had a head injury should be asked about neck pain, weakness, or paraesthesia in the upper and lower limbs. In the light of the above statistics, patients who are not able to give a clear history by virtue of altered consciousness should be assumed to have had a cervical spine injury until proven otherwise and should be handled accordingly.

Immediate immobilization of the cervical spine

If there are grounds to suspect that an accident victim might have sustained an injury of the cervical spine, every effort must be made to immobilise the cervical spine before the patient is moved at the scene of the accident (Box 7.1). This is best achieved by using a hard cervical collar that can be applied in two pieces and secured by Velcro strapping. Soft collars are not suitable as they provide little restriction of movement and because they are applied directly to the neck. Ideally, the collar should make contact above with the chin and the occiput and below with the sternum and the shoulders. This sort of collar stands away from the soft tissues of the neck. Collars that are applied directly to the neck may cause compression of the jugular veins and reduce the venous return from the head. This, in turn, may cause elevation of the intracranial pressure and, in the unconscious patient who is unable to protest, the exacerbation of already raised intracranial pressure may have a critical effect on the existing brain injury. A variety of well-designed collars are in common use.

When the head-injured patient is moved, the head and neck must be controlled. Ideally, three people are required to lift the patient without manipulation of the neck while a fourth individual takes charge of the head and neck (Fig. 7.1).

Once the patient has been placed on an ambulance trolley, he/she should remain there and as little movement of the spine as possible should be allowed until the integrity of the cervical spine has been established. If the patient must be moved from an ambulance trolley the same care should be exercised. Patients should not, however, because of concern about spinal injuries, be left lying on hard surfaces and in one position for periods of time. Only a matter of hours of immobility on a hard surface is required to cause skin necrosis and pressure sores. It is valuable to make an early judgement about the integrity of the spine in order to aid subsequent nursing care.

Box 7.1   Immediate management of cervical spine injury

- Suspect a cervical spine injury
- Apply a rigid collar
- Apply in-line traction when moving
- Use four-man lift
- Retain collar until spinal injury excluded

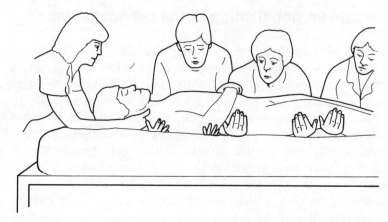

Fig. 7.1   The three-person lift also showing the fourth person stabilizing the head and neck.

Clinical assessment of spinal injury

Once the airway has been cleared, and respiration and blood volume have been stabilized, X-rays of the cervical spine should be obtained without moving the patient from the examination trolley. Anteroposterior, lateral, and open-mouth odontoid views of the cervical spine are required. If these X-rays are normal an unstable injury of the cervical spine is unlikely but cannot be excluded altogether and care must still be exercised in moving the patient and when passing an endotracheal tube.

History and examination

If the patient is conscious ask about pain in the neck and upper limbs. Ask about paraesthesia and weakness in the upper and lower limbs and establish when the patient last emptied the bladder. If the patient is unconscious ask witnesses whether the patient was seen to move all four limbs at the scene of the accident. The mechanism of the accident may also increase suspicion of a spinal injury. Falls from a height, high-velocity impacts, and falls from bicycles or horses, for instance, have a higher association with cervical spine injuries than blows to the head in assaults. The occupants of vehicles struck from behind commonly complain of neck pain which may be very persistent and troublesome despite normal imaging investigations.

On inspection, look for signs that indicate the mechanism of injury. Injuries to the face suggest the possibility of a hyperextension injury. Persistent rotation of the neck indicates the possibility of a unliateral facet dislocation. Observe spontaneous movement of the limbs in the unconscious patient. Priapism is associated with major spinal cord injury. Patients with high spinal cord injuries retaining only proximal upper limb power may lie with the upper limbs in flexion. Complete spinal cord injury may be accompanied by loss of vasomotor tone and hypotension. Lower cervical spinal cord injuries can result in paralysis of the muscles of respiration while sparing the innervation of the diaphragm so that the patient breathes only with the diaphragm. The chest fails to expand but the abdomen rises and falls with the respiratory effort.

Neurological examination

Examine the power in the upper and lower limbs in the conscious patient. Power can be graded using the Medical Research Council (MRC) scale shown in Box 7.2. Power should be examined in each major muscle group in turn and the results documented so that later deterioration can be recognized. The tendon reflexes should also be examined. Complete spinal cord injuries are accompanied by loss of the tendon reflexes in the acute stages as part of the phenomenon of spinal shock. Sensation should be tested in a systematic fashion, working from the scalp to the perineum. Remember that the lowest dermatomes—sacral dermatomes— are in the perianal area and the perineum (Fig. 7.2). Sensation should be tested using a safety pin, not a venepuncture needle, and the patient should indicate any change in the quality of the sensation. In a partial spinal cord injury there may be a change in the quality of the sensation from sharp to blunt at the level of the lesion. Very occasionally, the spinal cord injury is mostly unilateral and affects the pyramidal tract and spinothalamic tract in one half of the cord with the result that there may be weakness of the ipsilateral limbs but loss of pain and temperature sensation on the opposite side—a Brown–Sequaard lesion. When a patient

Box 7.2 MRC scale for muscle power

Grade	Muscle power
0	No muscle contraction
1	Muscle contraction only
2	Limb movement with gravity neutralized
3	Limb movement against gravity
4	Limb movement against added resistance
5	Normal power

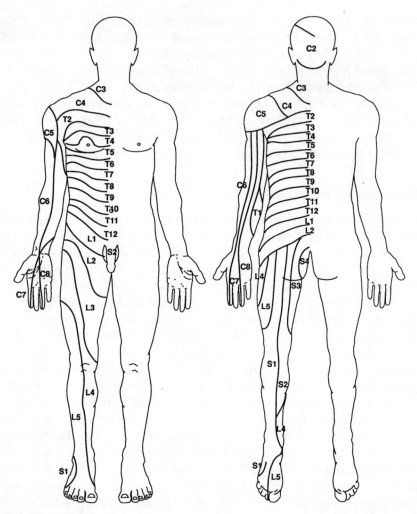

Fig. 7.2 Dermatome charts.

shows weakness only on one side, therefore, it is important to test sensation carefully on the opposite side of the body.

In the unconscious patient, observe spontaneous movements of the limbs or the limb movements evoked by a painful stimulus. Unconscious head-injured patients usually make some limb movement in response to a painful stimulus. No response to pain should raise the possibility of a high cervical spinal cord injury.

After resuscitation and neurological examination the unconscious patient must be log-rolled in order to allow inspection of the whole spine, looking for bruising, 'steps', or swelling. Log-rolling must be carried out by four people with one delegated to control the head and neck.

Investigation of spinal injuries

All unconscious patients with head injuries must be assumed to have had an injury of the cervical spine. In the fully conscious patient it is very unusual for an injury of the cervical spine to be completely asymptomatic and, in the absence of symptoms, it is reasonable not to request X-rays of the cervical spine. Multiply injured patients, however, may be conscious but so distracted by other injuries that symptoms of the cervical spine injury are not noticed and such patients should have X-rays of the cervical spine carried out.

Cervical spine X-rays should be among the early investigations in the head-injured patient. The doctor should insist on seeing lateral views of the whole of the cervical spine and should not accept views that do not include the C7/T1 junction. Lateral views of the lower cervical spine may be obtained more easily if traction is applied to the upper limbs or by use of the "swimmer's view", in which one arm is raised above the patient's head. Alternatively, a computerized tomography (CT) scan can be used to obtain images of the lower cervical vertebrae.

Remember that the absence of a fracture or misalignment on the initial X-rays does not necessarily mean that there is no spinal injury. In ligamentous injuries, there may be no loss of alignment while the patient lies with the neck in a neutral position. In the cooperative patient with neck pain the stability of the spine can be confirmed by carrying out further lateral views of the cervical spine with the neck in flexion and extension. This assessment must be postponed in the unconscious patient. Flexion and extension views may be prevented by neck muscle spasm. They should be carried out under the supervision of a doctor and stopped if any neurological symptoms develop.

Apparently normal X-rays of the cervical spine do not exclude an undisplaced, unstable ligamentous injury

---

When a fracture of the cervical spine is recognized, further imaging by CT may be helpful in order to define the configuration and extent of the fracture and its stability.

Interpretation of the radiology of the cervical spine is fully discussed in Chapter 5.

Early management of spine injuries

The patient with a suspected or confirmed cervical spine injury requires some form of immobilization of the neck. During resuscitation, this means the application of a suitable hard collar together with in-line manual traction when the patient is being moved. It is highly unlikely that additional neurological damage will occur during resuscitation and transfer if these simple measures are adhered to. Subsequent management will depend on the nature of the injury and the degree of instability. Further steps to immobilize the unstable cervical spine injury may be required but these are usually the responsibility of the specialist unit dealing with spinal injuries. In exceptional circumstances, if transfer to a specialist centre is delayed, seriously unstable cervical spine injuries should be treated with skull traction prior to transfer.

Skull traction

A variety of skull traction tongs are available but the most convenient, reliable, and easily applied by an experienced person are the Gardener–Wells tongs (Fig. 7.3). The scalp and periosteum are infiltrated with local anaesthetic at the widest part of the skull 2–3 cm above the ears. The pins of the traction tongs are screwed into the skull. The correct tension is indicated by a small stop that protrudes from the hub of one of the pins. When this stands out to 2 mm the tension is correct. A cord is then attached to the tongs and passed over a pulley on the head of the bed. Weights are then attached to the cord so that traction is applied in the line of the neck. The weight applied depends on the level of the injury. A useful guide in adults is to apply 5 lb (2.2 kg) for each vertebra from the atlas downwards. Thus, for example, for a fracture/dislocation at the C5/C6 level traction of 25–30 lb (11–13 kg) would be required.

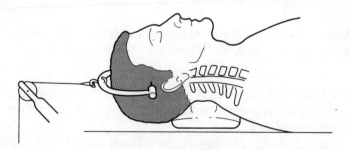

Fig. 7.3   The application of Gardner–Wells tongs.

Traction is applied gradually by increasing the weight in stages, with X-rays at intervals to ensure that the spine is not being overdistracted.

Nursing the patient in traction

The patient in skull traction must not be able to move in the bed and is at risk, from an early stage, of developing skin necrosis from pressure. It is essential to turn the patient at 2-hourly intervals to prevent pressure sores. This requires a suitable bed and the choice is influenced by whether or not the patient has a spinal cord injury and is paraplegic. If the patient is paraplegic the ideal arrangement is some form of tilting bed such as the Stoke Mandeville or Egerton bed which allow the patient to be tilted from side-to-side in traction. If necessary, when a special bed is not available, an ordinary hospital bed can be used as a temporary measure. The patient can be tilted by placing pillows under one side of the mattress in order to tilt the patient from side-to-side. In the case of a patient with a seriously unstable cervical spine injury who is not paraplegic, care must be taken that the patient does not move around the bed while the head is fixed by traction. An alternative to the arrangements described above is the Stryker frame which allows the patient to be turned from prone to supine at intervals. This requires some experience to apply and it can be difficult to manage a restless patient in this fashion. Whatever arrangement is used, it is important that anxiety about spinal instability does not prevent the patient from being turned regularly.

Immobile patients with spinal injuries must be turned regularly to prevent skin necrosis

---

Stability and instability

Cervical spine fractures are classified according to the anatomical level and the mechanism of injury. In each case, the most important factor influencing the patient's management is the stability of the injury and the possibility of progressive loss of alignment. The main role of surgery in the management of cervical spine injury is to ensure stability.

Types of cervical spine injury

Fractures of the upper cervical spine differ from those from C3 to C7 because of the peculiar anatomy of the upper two vertebrae. (See also Box 7.3 which shows the classification of cervical spine injury.)

Box 7.3 Classification of cervical spine injury

- Fractures of atlas C1
- Fractures of axis C2   – Odontoid fractures
                                      – Hangman's fractures
- Injuries of   C3–C7 – Flexion
                                      – Flexion rotation
                                      – Extension of normal spine
                                      – Extension of spondylotic spine
                                      – Compression
- Cervical cord concussion

Fractures of the atlas: C1

Fractures of the ring of the atlas (Jefferson fractures) are uncommon and are usually caused by compression, as in a fall from a height or by hyper-extension of the neck. Neurological damage is unusual and these fractures are relatively stable and can be managed by a brace or well-fitting hard collar.

Fractures of the axis: C2

Fractures of C2 fall into two groups: (1) fractures of the ring of C2 (hangman's fractures, Fig. 7.4); and (2) fractures of the odontoid process. Because of the width of the spinal canal at this level, spinal cord injury is

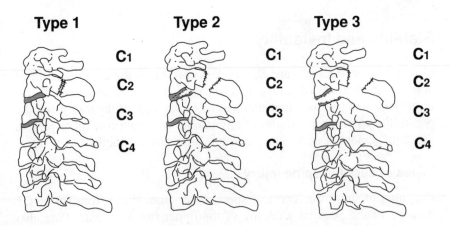

Fig. 7.4 Hangman's (C2) fractures.

not common as a result of these fractures. The stability of the hangman's fracture depends on its configuration and this may not be clear until detailed images are obtained by CT. These injuries can usually be managed conservatively in a cervical brace.

Fractures of the odontoid process (Fig. 7.5) are unstable and can be complicated by progressive displacement and spinal cord injury. They are classified according to the level at which the fracture transects the process. Fractures through the body of C2 (type 3) have a broad base and, if not displaced, can be treated conservatively with a cervical brace or halo fixation device. Fractures at the junction of the odontoid and the vertebral body (type 2) have a smaller fracture surface and are less likely to remain undisplaced or to unite. The same is true of fractures through

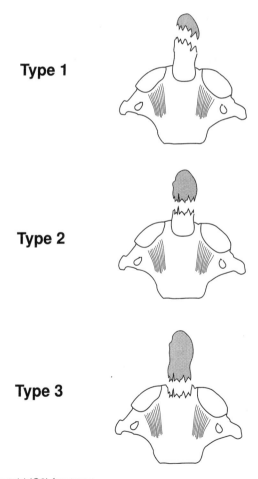

Type 1

Type 2

Type 3

Fig. 7.5 Odontoid (C2) fractures.

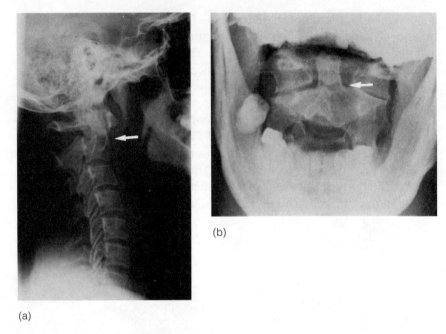

(b)

(a)

Fig. 7.6 Lateral (a) and open-mouth (b) fractures.

the mid portion of the odontoid (type 1) and these fractures are more likely to require some form of surgical stabilization.

On X-rays of the cervical spine odontoid fractures (Fig. 7.6) are easily missed. Good quality antero-posterior and lateral views are required. In the conscious patient an antero-posterior view through the open mouth should be obtained. Note that, even although the fracture itself may not be easily seen on the antero-posterior view, the odontoid process may be seen to be displaced laterally.

Failure to recognize these unstable fractures may lead to progressive displacement and eventual high spinal cord injury.

Fractures and dislocations of the lower cervical spine

The most practical classification of injuries of the cervical spine below C2 is based on the mechanism of injury. These injuries are the result of flexion, extension, rotation, axial compression, or a combination of these forces (Fig. 7.7). Stability depends on the mechanism of injury and the configuration of the damage to bone or ligaments.

In the lower cervical spine, the commonest injuries are those caused by flexion. These injuries are seen following road traffic accidents and

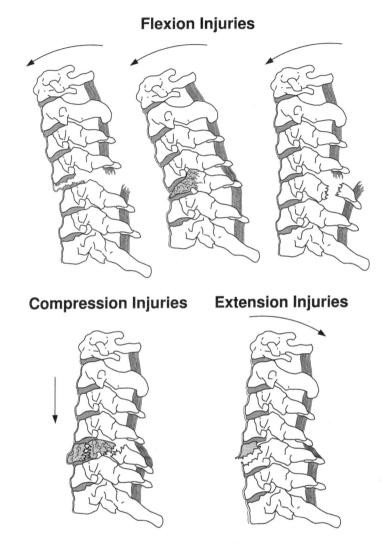

Fig. 7.7 Mechanisms of lower cervical spine injuries.

falls from bicycles or horses. If the ligaments remain intact there may simply be wedging of the anterior aspect of the vertebral body (Fig. 7.8). This type of injury is likely to be stable and may be treated conservatively with repeat X-rays at intervals. On the other hand, flexion may cause bony injury or disruption of ligaments resulting in potential or actual loss of alignment (Fig. 7.9). These injuries require reduction of the dislocation and stabilization—often by surgery.

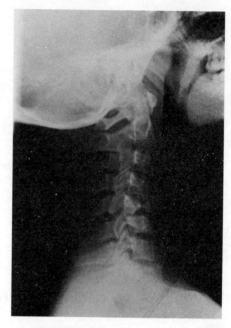

Fig. 7.8   Lateral cervical spine X-ray. Fracture caused by flexion and axial compression.

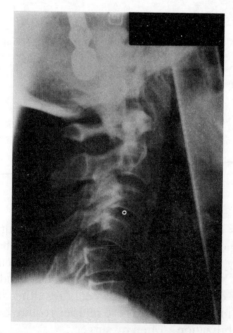

Fig. 7.9   Unstable flexion injury with dislocation at C4/C5.

Hyperextension injuries of the cervical spine are less common than flexion injuries. They are often caused by falling or by road traffic accidents. The fact that the patient has evidence of facial injuries should draw attention to the possible extension injury of cervical spine. Hyperextension may cause disruption of the anterior longitudinal ligament of the spine with widening of the disc space anteriorly. There may be avulsion of the anterior margin of one vertebral body. This injury can result in instability but it can usually be managed conservatively by preventing further extension of the neck with a good collar or a brace.

Flexion and extension may each cause disruption of ligaments alone, resulting in instability, subluxation or even complete dislocation. The combination of flexion and rotation may cause dislocation of one facet joint. When there has been a ligamentous injury only the first X-rays may show no displacement but progressive subluxation can take place over succeeding weeks. The possibility of potential ligamentous instability should be considered if there is a history of violent flexion or if there is an increased anterior spinal soft tissue shadow (Fig. 5.11). Patients with even a very minor degree of misalignment who are treated in a collar or brace should have regular X-rays carried out to detect progressive subluxation. Whereas fractures are expected to heal if immobilized, ligamentous injuries are more likely to remain unstable and often require surgical stabilization.

Extension injuries of the spondylotic spine

Spinal cord damage can take place without instability of the spine. A direct blow can cause a spinal cord contusion with no radiological abnormality. More commonly, spinal cord injuries can occur as a result of hyperextension of the spondylotic cervical spine. In patients with cervical spondylosis the spinal canal is narrow because of osteophyte formation. Hyperextension further narrows the spinal canal, resulting in transient compression of the spinal cord. The relatively avascular centre of the cord is rendered ischaemic while the more superficial parts are spared. Since the upper limbs are represented more centrally in the spinal cord there may be more obvious weakness in the upper limbs than in the legs. This injury is seen most commonly in older patients who have fallen and who often have coexisting facial injuries. X-rays show features of cervical spondylosis but no fracture or dislocation. Surgical treatment is not indicated and treatment is confined to rehabilitation and restriction of neck movement with a collar.

Surgical management of cervical spine injuries

Immediate surgical intervention is rarely indicated in injuries of the cervical spine. Alignment can usually be restored by traction, if necessary, and stability ensured by the use of the traction or an external brace or collar in the first instance. If, however, traction fails to reduce a cervical dislocation because of either unilateral or bilateral facet joint dislocation (locked facets), open reduction may be required. This situation usually occurs if there has been a delay in admission or diagnosis. If alignment has been restored and the cervical spine has been immobilized surgical stabilization can be arranged as an elective procedure.

A detailed discussion of the surgical management of cervical spine injuries is beyond the scope of this book. The reader should be aware of the problem of spinal instability and be prepared to seek specialist advice when there is any clinical or radiological suspicion of instability.

Limiting further spinal cord damage

The injured spinal cord is vulnerable to further insults, much in the same way as the brain. The principal means of preventing further damage is to ensure stability of the spine from the time of admission (Box 7.4). As in the case of brain injuries, hypoxia, hypotension, and anaemia may cause further neurological damage and the patient with a spinal cord injury requires close monitoring. A high spinal cord injury may be the reason for respiratory impairment. Oxygen saturation monitoring and blood gas analysis should be used to detect respiratory impairment in the patient with a cervical cord lesion. The loss of vasomotor tone caused by a spinal cord injury may result in hypotension. Blood pressure monitoring, intravenous fluid replacement, and monitoring of urine output are essential parts of the early management of spinal cord injuries.

There have been reports that spinal cord damage can be limited by high-dose corticosteroids, **naloxone**, and by cooling. The role of these

---

Box 7.4   Limiting further cord damage

- Immobilization of the cervical spine
- Adequate oxygenation
- Prevention of hypotension
- Correction of anaemia

techniques remains uncertain and, as yet, no clear evidence from clinical trials supports their routine use.

Complications of spinal cord injury

A number of medical complications occur in patients with spinal cord injury and, to a lesser extent, in those who are immobilized in bed after spinal injuries without cord damage (Box 7.5). These complications are due to immobility, impairment of autonomic function, and respiratory insufficiency and can be both anticipated and prevented.

Deep venous thrombosis

Immobility and the increase in blood coagulability that follows trauma expose the patient to the risk of deep venous thrombosis (DVT). The risk of DVT in patients with spinal cord injury has been estimated to be approximately 10% in one series of 1500 patients. If the patient is to be immobilized prophylactic measures must be taken to prevent DVT. Low-dose subcutaneous **heparin** (5000 units twice daily) and thromboembolic stockings are commonly used for this purpose.

Pressure sores

Skin ischaemia can develop within hours in the immobile patient, leading to ulceration that may require long and tedious treatment. This condition is much easier to prevent than to treat and prophylactic measures must be initiated as soon as the patient is admitted to hospital. If the patient is unable to move, his/her position must be manually changed every two hours, or use a suitable bed. During periods of immobility the pressure areas can be protected by sheepskin padding, water-filled balloons, or by lacing the patient on special mattresses. The uninitiated are often

---

Box 7.5 Medical complications of spinal injury

- Deep venous thrombosis
- Pressure sores
- Chest infection
- Bradycardia
- Hypotension
- Hypothermia
- Urinary tract infection

anxious about moving the patient with head or spinal injuries but this is an essential part of the early management.

Chest infection

A variety of factors conspire to cause chest infections in patients with spinal injuries. First, if the spinal cord is injured there may be weakness of the muscles of respiration. This may not be apparent at the time of admission but can begin to have an adverse effect as the patient tires or because of sedative drugs and the supine position. The key to early recognition of this problem is careful monitoring of respiratory function.

Autonomic complications

Cervical cord injuries may result in interruption of the sympathetic outflow. The vagus may be unopposed and this can result in brady-arrhythmias. The loss of sympathetic tone also causes peripheral vaso-dilatation and hypotension. Such patients may become hypertensive while lying down but they are particularly inclined to postural hypo-tension. Adequate fluid replacement reduces the impact of autonomic impairment. Immobility and peripheral vasodilatation both contribute to hypothermia, particularly in patients who may have spent some hours in the resuscitation room. Efforts should be made to prevent heat loss during resuscitation.

Urinary tract infection

Patients with spinal cord injury will commonly require catheterization of the bladder in the early stages of treatment and are therefore exposed to the risk of urinary tract infection. The paraplegic patient will be able to localize the attendant discomfort and may react by sweating, becoming pyrexial, vomiting, or developing a tachycardia.

Delayed complications of spinal injury

Delayed subluxation

Potential instability of the cervical spine may not be recognized in the early X-rays if the spine remains in normal alignment. If there has been disruption of the ligaments there may be delayed subluxation and the patient may return, complaining of neck pain or of neurological symptoms in the limbs. X-rays of the cervical spine should be repeated. Because there can be difficulty obtaining adequate views of the C7/T1 area missed subluxations are commonly at this level.

Cervical disc prolapse

Cervical spine injury may be complicated by cervical disc prolapse. The patient may have had neck pain after the injury and then returns with neurological symptoms in the limbs. A central disc prolapse will cause progressive disturbance of gait, altered sensation in the lower limbs and paraesthesia, and motor disturbance in the upper limbs. Alternatively, a postero-lateral disc prolapse may present with arm pain and paraesthesia, together with neurological signs suggesting a nerve root lesion.

Plain X-rays in patients with cervical disc prolapse may show narrowing of a single disc space and a loss of the normal cervical lordosis. Confirmation of a cervical disc prolapse requires either magnetic resonance imaging (MRI) or a cervical myelogram. CT scanning is not suitable.

Central cervical disc prolapse requires early surgical treatment. Initially, the patient with a postero-lateral disc prolapse and arm pain can be managed conservatively, using traction, collars, and antiinflammatory analgesics. Persistent pain calls for surgical intervention.

Whiplash syndrome

This is a common syndrome in victims of road traffic accidents and it rarely occurs after other forms of trauma. The patient is the occupant of a vehicle that has been struck from behind. The neck is abruptly hyper-extended and there may be immediate pain in the neck. More commonly, however, there is a delay before the patient presents with neck pain. X-rays of the cervical spine show no evidence of fracture or subluxation. Neck pain becomes persistent and may be accompanied by headache. Patients frequently fail to return to work because of the symptoms. There is no history of arm pain or numbness or weakness in the upper limbs which might suggest a cervical disc prolapse.

On examination, neck movements may be restricted but there are no abnormal neurological signs. Imaging investigations are normal. It is a feature of this condition that the severity of the symptoms is in striking contrast to the minimal physical and radiological findings.

The pathological basis of this syndrome remains unknown. Given the circumstances of the injury, it is likely that psychological factors play a part in some patients. The patient is usually the innocent party in an accident. Resolution of legal and insurance issues can be slow and cause anxiety and frustration. Alarming accidents can be the cause of post-traumatic neurosis (post-traumatic stress syndrome). In some patients the symptoms settle following the conclusion of litigation. In many, however, there is undoubtedly an organic basis for these very persistent symptoms. Extensive investigations are not helpful once the patient has been shown to have no neurological deficit and no unstable spinal injury. Sophisticated investigations, such as MRI or myelography are not indicated.

Management of this syndrome requires, first, positive exclusion of a previously missed subluxation or cervical disc prolapse. The patient should be reassured that no serious damage has taken place. In the immediate aftermath of the injury severe neck pain can be relieved by a hard cervical collar and analgesics. Long-term use of collars should be discouraged and the patient should be encouraged to dispense with the collar and move the neck as soon as the severe pain has settled. This may require the help of a physiotherapist. When neck pain persists for months and the patient seeks repeated medical advice it is necessary to consider the possibility that the patient may be depressed or suffering from an anxiety neurosis. It is useful to make detailed notes of the history of injury, the initial treatment, and the radiological findings because the majority of these injuries will eventually become the subject of litigation or insurance claims.

Further reading

Meyer P. R. (1989). *Surgery of spine trauma*. Churchill Livingstone, New York.
Shrago G. G. (1973). Cervical spine injuries associated with head trauma: review of 50 patients. *American Journal of Radiology*, **118**, 670–3.
Grundy, D., Swain, A. (1996). ABC of Spinal Cord Injury. *British Medical Journal*.

8 *Head injuries in children*

Chapter contents

Key points in head injuries in children

1 In Britain, falling is estimated to cause 40–50% of head injury in children.

2 The commonest cause of severe head injury in children is their running into the paths of oncoming vehicles.

3 In children subjected to physical abuse the commonest cause of death is head injury.

4 A head injury caused by shaking may present no outward sign of head trauma, but may be accompanied by a history of vomiting, fits, failure to thrive, lassitude, and irritability.

5 Where there is a history of trauma suspicion may be raised by an account inconsistent with the physical findings, the vagueness of the history, or an undue delay in seeking medical advice. Also by evidence of multiple injuries of different ages, or of neglect, and characteristic types of lesion: retinal haemorrhages, bruising in a fingertip pattern, and cigarette burns.

6 Radiologically, complex or multiple fractures, fractures involving more than one bone, and occipital fractures are suggestive of non-accidental injury, as are wide or 'growing' fractures and acute subdural and intracerebral haematomas and haemorrhagic contusion in the absence of skull fractures.

7 If a non-accidental cause is suspected the child must be admitted and an urgent consultation with a consultant paediatrician should be arranged.

8 In children under five conscious level should be assessed on the Glasgow Paediatric Coma Scale.

9 A 'growing fracture' (normally found in children under 3 years) requires surgical repair in order to prevent the development of a skull defect that might render the underlying brain liable to injury.

10 *Contre-coup* cerebral contusions are rare in children, and should raise the possibility of non-accidental injury.

11 It is vital that information on the progress of a child with head injury is given to the parents consistently by a single senior person who is identified as being 'in charge'.

Head injuries in children

The epidemiology of head injury in children differs from that in adults, and the head injury in the child poses special problems of diagnosis, management, and rehabilitation.

The widespread belief that children, having youth on their side, are more able to tolerate and recover from head injuries than adults is erroneous. The developing brain is especially vulnerable to injury. On the other hand, children are less frequently injured as occupants of vehicles involved in road traffic accidents, and thus tend to avoid the high-velocity head injuries so commonly seen in adults.

For the parents, the trauma of the child's injury is compounded by feelings of guilt, remorse, and anger. Since the parents may spend much of their time by the bedside of the injured child, other children in the family may be relatively neglected at a time when they most need reassurance.

Causes of head injuries in children

The commonest cause of head injury in children is falling, estimated in various surveys in Britain as 40–50% of children's head injuries. Falls occur in the domestic situation and at play. In infants, falling from chairs or changing tables is a frequent variety of accident. The incident is commonly not witnessed, and there is uncertainty whether the child had really fallen or not. Accidents at play are also often unwitnessed by adults, since they may occur out of doors, and the nature and severity of the blow is not known. Although domestic falls are common, and cause parents a good deal of anguish, they do not often result in severe head injuries. Resulting skull fractures from these mechanisms are usually closed linear fractures, and subsequent intracranial haematomas are uncommon. (See Box 8.1.)

Approximately 20% of rear seat occupants in Britain are children. Children are involved as passengers in road traffic accidents, and their situation in the back seat does not diminish the possible severity of the trauma—indeed, there is evidence that rear seat passengers suffer more severe injuries than belted front seat passengers. A study in the United States has shown an incidence of head injury of 70% in children involved

Box 8.1   Causes of head injury in children

- Falls
- Road-traffic accidents
- Sports injuries
- Non-accidental injury

as rear seat passengers in road traffic accidents. It was estimated that the use of rear seat belts could bring about a reduction of deaths in rear seat passengers of 75%. The now compulsory use of seat belts in the rear seats is expected to reduce severe injuries from this source. Children under the age of 4 years should be restrained in safety seats. Children over the age of 4 can be protected by standard seat belts as long as a suitable booster cushion is used.

The commonest source of severe head injuries in children in their running out in front of vehicles as pedestrians. Children as young as 4 or 5 years are regular victims, and lack of parental supervision plays an important part in the circumstances. These children suffer multiple injuries.

A British survey in 1991 found that 36% of head injuries in children were due to road traffic accidents.

Bicycle accidents are another common cause of head injury, and one which can also be reduced by safety measures such as the use of cycle helmets, the provision of cycle tracks, and the provision of cycling proficiency courses in schools. These head injuries are associated particularly with injuries of the cervical spine, upper limbs, and clavicles.

Non-accidental injury

It is important to be aware of the possibility that the injured child may be the victim of abuse. By its nature, the true incidence of this phenomenon is difficult to determine. One recent survey in England found that only 4% of all head injuries in children were due to non-accidental injury.

In children subjected to physical abuse, the commonest cause of death is head injury. If the injury is caused by shaking there may be no outward sign of head trauma. In these circumstances the child may present with a history of vomiting, fits, failure to thrive, lassitude, and irritability. Where there is a history of trauma suspicion may be raised by an account inconsistent with the physical findings, the vagueness of the history, or an undue delay in seeking medical advice. On physical examination there may be evidence of multiple injuries of different ages, the child may appear neglected, or the child's affect may be abnormal—withdrawn, frightened, or depressed. Retinal haemorrhages do not occur as a result of simple falls, and are well-recognized in association with non-accidental head injuries. Certain skin lesions are characteristic of physical abuse, and these include fingertip bruising (i.e. fingertip pressure) and cigarette burns.

Be aware of the possibility of non-accidental injury

Box 8.2   Clinical features of non-accidental injury

- History inconsistent with physical findings
- Vague account of accident
- Delay in seeking medical attention
- Multiple injuries
- Child with abnormal affect
- Signs of neglect
- Characteristic skin lesions
- Retinal haemorrhages

Certain radiological features increase the suspicion of non-accidental injury. Complex or multiple fractures, fractures involving more than one bone, and occipital fractures are highly suggestive. It has also been reported that wide or 'growing' fractures are characteristics of non-accidental head injury (see p. 126). Skull fractures in children, as in adults, may be complicated by extradural haemorrhage; but in the non-accidental injury subdural haematomas, intracerebral haematomas, and haemorrhagic contusion are common causes of neurological impairment and death. These lesions are often due to shaking, and may be found in the absence of a skull fracture. Their finding should raise the possibility of non-accidental injury. (See Box 8.2.)

If a non-accidental cause for the head injury is considered the child must be admitted to hospital, and urgent consultation with a consultant paediatrician should be arranged. A skeletal survey should be carried out in order to identify other injuries.

Clinical assessment of the head-injured child

Glasgow Paediatric Coma Scale

Exactly the same priorities apply to the resuscitation of the injured child as have been described for the adult. The neurological assessment, however, is complicated by difficulties of communication and co-operation in the younger child. In children over the age of 5 the adult Glasgow Coma Scale (see Box 1.3) can be used to describe conscious level. In younger children the recording of the verbal response must be modified, and in children too young to be able to obey a command the 'motor response' element must be modified accordingly. The **Glasgow Pediatric Coma Scale** has been devised (Box 8.3).

Box 8.3   Glasgow Paediatric Coma Scale

		> *1 year*	< *1 year*	
Eye-opening response	4	spontaneously	spontaneously	
	3	to command	to shout	
	2	to pain	to pain	
	1	no response	no response	
Best motor response	5	obeys commands		
	4	localizes pain	localizes pain	
	3	flexion to pain	flexion to pain	
	2	extension to pain	extension to pain	
	1	no response	no response	

		> *5 years*	*2–5 years*	*0–2 years*
Best verbal response	5	orientated and converses	appropriate words and phrases	smiles and cries appropriately
	4	disorientated and converses	inappropriate words	cries
	3	inappropriate words	cries	inappropriate crying
	2	incomprehensible sounds	grunting	grunting
	1	no response	no response	no response
Normal aggregate score			< 6 months	12
			6–12 months	12
			1–2 years	13
			2–5 years	14
			> 5 years	14

Radiological assessment

Linear skull fractures in children are no different from those seen in adults. In young children some fractures grow in width under the influence of raised intracranial pressure—in the presence of a subdural haematoma, for instance. (See Box 8.4.) The skull injury may involve unfused sutures, and present radiologically as a widened suture line.

Box 8.4 Radiological features of non-accidental injury

- Complex or multiple fractures
- Wide or growing fractures
- Occipital fractures
- Radiology inconsistent with history of injury
- Fractures of other bones and differing ages
- Subdural haematoma
- Cerebral contusion/intracerebral haematoma

Depressed skull fractures in the young child with a soft pliable skull may present as '**pond fractures**'—saucer-shaped depressions rather like an indentation in a table tennis ball. It may be difficult to gain the cooperation from a distressed or frightened child in order to obtain good quality skull X-rays. It may be necessary to admit the child and defer further investigation until the child's confidence has been gained. The presence of a parent during the X-ray may be helpful. Because of the potential difficulties in obtaining a reliable history there should be a lower threshold for ordering skull X-rays in children.

The indications for computerized tomography (CT) scanning are the same as for adults; but it may be impossible to obtain a satisfactory scan in the restless or disturbed child. If the clinical indications are pressing, the child will require a general anaesthetic in order to carry out the scan.

Scalp injuries

The capacity for scalp lacerations to bleed heavily presents a potentially serious problem in small children, who can lose a significant proportion of their total blood volume from this source. Bleeding may also take place into the plane between the galea and the pericranium. The **subgaleal haematoma** forms a tense swelling extending from the forehead to the occiput. This may be extremely painful, and presents an alarming appearance. In the small child it may represent a significant loss of circulating blood volume. Unless aspiration of the haematoma is essential for pain relief no specific treatment is required, and the haematoma will resolve spontaneously. Aspiration carries the risk of introducing infection—potentially serious infection, with infarction of part of the scalp— and should be carried out with meticulous asepsis.

Skull fractures

Children's skulls are more pliable than those of adults, and may be deformed to a greater extent without fracturing. Linear fractures carry the same implications in children as they do in adults. The **pond fracture** referred to above may be disfiguring if it is outside the hairline, but requires no treatment if it is within the hairline and not associated with an overlying wound. The parents will need to be reassured that the palpable dent is harmless and will eventually disappear. If the fracture poses a cosmetic problem it is a simple matter to elevate the depressed portion of skull.

In a small proportion of young children with linear skull fractures there is a tendency for the fracture to grow. This phenomenon is rarely seen over the age of 3 years. As the fracture edges become more widely separated a skull defect is created. These are known as **growing fractures**. The reasons for this complication remain uncertain, but it is thought that it may be related to an underlying dural tear which allows herniation of arachnoid into the fracture. A growing fracture requires surgical repair in order to prevent the development of a skull defect which might render the underlying brain vulnerable to injury. The defect is explored and the underlying dural defect repaired. The fracture is repaired with a bone graft. In order to recognize this problem all children under the age of 3 years with substantial skull fractures should be reviewed as outpatients after about three months. Clinical examination of the fracture site is sufficient to exclude a skull defect, and only those with a clinical suspicion of a growing fracture need be X-rayed.

Children with large skull fractures should be reviewed after three months to exclude growing fracture

---

Paediatric concussion syndrome

A peculiar feature of concussional injuries in children is the alarming deterioration that can take place within a short time of a relatively minor concussional injury. Typically, the child suffers a concussional injury but recovers consciousness and has a lucid interval during which he/she is able to speak. There is then a deterioration in consciousness, often associated with extreme restlessness. The pattern is indistinguishable from that seen in the patient with a developing extradural haematoma and the patient must be managed accordingly until an intracranial haematoma has been excluded. The child may be so restless that a CT scan cannot be carried out without a general anaesthetic. When the scan shows no evidence of an intracranial mass ventilation is not required and the condition recovers within 24 hours in most cases.

This syndrome is thought to be due to hyperaemia and swelling of the child's brain as a reaction to trauma and seems to run a benign course with appropriate nursing alone.

Intracranial haematomas in children

Extradural haematomas are seen in children, and present in the same clinical fashion as in adults. Whereas, in adults, 80% of extradural haematomas are associated with a skull fracture seen on the skull X-ray, the incidence of associated skull fractures is lower in children—in the region of 60%. This may be related to the greater elasticity of the child's skull and the greater adherence of the dura to the suture lines. Management of the child with a suspected extradural haematoma is no different from that in the adult; but there must be a greater readiness to admit the child with a head injury for observation, since one important indication of the possibility of extradural haematoma—the skull fracture—may be absent.

> **Children should be admitted for observation even in the absence of a skull fracture after significant head injuries**

Acute subdural haematomas are not common in children, and should raise the possibility of non-accidental injury. **Chronic subdural haematomas** are sometimes seen, and are most common in children under the age of three years. In many instances, a history of trauma is not obtained, and the haematoma may be due to a relatively minor injury which has passed unnoticed. The history is usually one of irritability, vomiting, disturbed sleep and feeding patterns, and drowsiness and these children are less likely to present primarily to an A&E department.

Contre-coup cerebral contusions are rarely seen in children, and, again, should raise the possibility of non-accidental injury.

Management of head-injured children

Head-injured children are more likely than adults to be admitted to non-specialist units for observation. In many instances, this will mean admission to a children's hospital separate from the adult hospital and the neurosurgical department. An adult with the same injury might be considered worthy of admission to the neurosurgical ward under the care of medical staff, and, more importantly, nursing staff, with specialist experience in the observation and management of the unconscious patient. The role of experienced neurosurgical nurses should not be underestimated, and there is a strong case for insisting that children with potentially serious head injuries should be observed in the early period of the illness in the neurosurgical ward.

The parents are also patients

The experience of having a child with a severe head injury is both terrifying and very distressing for the parents. Most parents will wish to remain in the hospital and at the bed-side during the critical period. They will repeatedly seek reassurance from the medical and nursing staff, and from the physiotherapists and members of other disciplines, that their child is going to make a full recovery. At this stage, every hint of progress or deterioration is seized; and it is vital that consistent information is given by one person, who is identified as being 'in charge'. This should be a senior member of staff. Apparent discrepancies in the information given increase the anxiety and, however unintentionally, give the impression that information is being concealed. In the case of the severe head injury, there are two stages to the process, and these should be explained to the parents. The first stage is the period when efforts are directed towards ensuring the child's survival; and at this stage it is usually impossible to give accurate information about the quality of recovery that might be expected. The second stage is the period of recovery and rehabilitation, during which the rate of recovery and the extent of possible recovery begin to become apparent. Care of the parents, the provision of simple factual information, and the availability of the doctor in charge of the child build a rapport that is essential in the long-term management of the head-injured child.

Further reading

Diagnosis and treatment of head injury in children. *In Neurological Surgery*, 4th edition, (ed. J. R. Youmans), vol. 3, W.B. Saunders, Philadelphia.

Becker, D. P. and Gudeman, S. K. (ed.) (1989). *Textbook of head injury*, (Chapter 15), Paediatric head injuries—special considerations. W. B. Saunders, Philadelphia.

Hobbs, C. J. (1989). ABC of child abuse—head injuries. *British Medical Journal*, **298**, 1169–70.

McLaurin, R. L. and Touban, R. (1996). Diagnosis and treatment of head injury in children. In *Neurological surgery*, 4th edition (ed. J. R. Youmans), Chapters 70/71. W. B. Saunders, Philadelphia.

9 Operative surgery

Chapter contents

Key points in operative surgery

1 It is important to shave the scalp sufficiently to give a clear view of the surgical field, and to enable the wound to be extended if necessary. Surgical wounds should be planned so that they can be incorporated in more extensive scalp flaps should further surgery prove necessary after transfer to a specialist unit.
2 Bleeding from the scalp and extradural space can be heavy, so if anything more than a minor procedure is planned blood should be cross-matched in preparation.
3 The great majority of scalp lacerations can be closed under local anaesthesia with 1% lignocaine and 1/200 000 adrenaline: but lengthy lacerations, scalping injuries and wounds involving skin loss should *not* be treated under local anaesthetic.
4 General anaesthetic technique should ensure that intracranial hypertension is not exacerbated during induction or in the course of surgery: the patient must be paralysed and ventilated, and *not* allowed to breathe spontaneously. Hypotension must be avoided so as to maintain adequate cerebral perfusion.
5 Once the patient is anaesthetized the endotracheal tube must be firmly anchored before the head is draped and the anaesthetist's access is obscured; the head should be supported on a head ring. A 30° head-up tilt of the operating table once the patient is anaesthetized helps to keep down intracranial pressure.
6 In ragged or contaminated scalp wounds care should be taken not to excise so much skin that the wound cannot be closed without tension.
7 In compound depressed skull fractures if the dura has been torn the laceration should be extended in order to inspect the brain and to remove foreign material, clot, and contaminated or devitalized tissue from it if necessary. Prophylactic antibiotics should be prescribed in all cases.

In Britain, it is usually possible and desirable for head-injured patients requiring operative intervention to be transferred to a specialist unit. There are occasions when circumstances make this impossible, and the general surgeon or orthopaedic surgeon may be required to operate in the district general hospital. Indeed, in many parts of the world the surgical management of head injuries is, of necessity, the responsibility of the general surgeon.

In this chapter, those procedures that may be necessary in non-specialist units are described. Modifications to routine neurosurgical practice have been made, on the assumption that available equipment will be limited. Certain basic instruments are essential, and should be stored together as a craniotomy set.

Before embarking on cranial surgery certain principles should be borne in mind. It is important to shave the scalp sufficiently to give a clear view of the surgical field, and to enable the wound to be extended if necessary. Surgical wounds should be planned so that they can be incorporated in more extensive scalp flaps if further surgery may be necessary after transfer to a specialist unit. Bleeding from the scalp and from the extradural space can be heavy, and, if anything more than a minor procedure is planned, blood should be cross-matched in preparation.

Anaesthesia

Local anaesthesia

The great majority of scalp lacerations can be closed under local anaesthesia using 1% lignocaine and adrenaline 1/200 000. Lengthy lacerations, scalping injuries, and wounds involving skin loss should not be treated under local anaesthetic, and these wounds should be cleaned and dressed and then left until the patient has been suitably resuscitated and prepared for a general anaesthetic.

General anaesthesia

The head-injured patient poses specific problems for the anaesthetist from the stage of resuscitation, during transfer, in the operating theatre, and in the intensive care unit. The anaesthetist must be familiar with the pathophysiology of head injury and the effects of anaesthetic technique on cerebral perfusion. These issues are discussed in Chapter 10.

Uncomplicated scalp laceration

Shave the scalp to give adequate exposure of the wound. Clean the surrounding skin with antiseptic solution and drape the area. Infiltrate the skin edges with local anaesthetic (but where there is any skin loss a large volume of injected local anaesthetic can hinder approximation of the wound edges). Retract the wound edges and inspect the underlying skull for fractures.

In ragged or contaminated wounds the wound edge should be excised sparingly, taking care not to excise so much skin that the wound cannot be closed without tension.

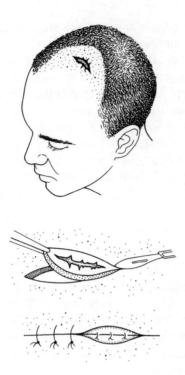

Fig. 9.1   Suture of a scalp wound.

Small wounds should be sutured in a single layer, using a non-absorbable suture material of gauge 3/0, such as nylon or silk or surgical staples. In large wounds, it is preferable to carry out a two-layer closure, approximating the galea with absorbable sutures such as Vicryl, Dexon, or PDS and lightly approximating the skin edges with interrupted non-absorbable sutures (see Fig. 9.1).

Compound depressed skull fracture

Widely shave the scalp around the wound and position the head in the head ring. Clean the skin with antiseptic solution, and drape the prepared area.

The wound is cautiously excised, taking care not to create a skin defect that cannot be closed without tension. Extend the wound in order to give a clear view of the fracture (Fig. 9.2). A self-retaining retractor is inserted, and, in small wounds, this will usually ensure haemostasis. In larger wounds haemostasis is achieved by picking up the galea in artery

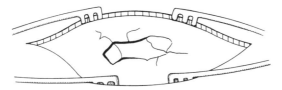

Fig. 9.2 Exposure of a depressed fracture.

forceps at 2–3 cm intervals and everting the skin edges. The artery forceps can be bunched together and retained by an elastic band.

Having exposed the fracture incise the pericranium. A periosteal elevator is used to scrape the pericranium from the margins of the fracture.

The depressed bone fragments must now be elevated in order that the underlying dura can be inspected. It may be possibly simply to lift out the fragments using bone rongeurs, but in many cases the depressed fragments are impacted. It is then necessary to fashion a burr hole on the edge of the fracture so that an instrument can be inserted under the fracture (Fig. 9.3).

Remove the bone fragments and clean them by washing in a solution of **flucloxacillin** (500 mg in 500 ml normal saline), and set them aside. Foreign material is removed from the skull defect.

If the dura has been torn the laceration should be extended in order to inspect the brain (Fig. 9.4). Remove foreign material from the cortical laceration. Clot and contaminated or devitalized brain are removed by gentle suction. Haemostasis can usually be secured by gentle packing with cotton-wool pledgets soaked in normal saline. Packing for 5–10 minutes is generally effective at controlling diffuse oozing. Alternatively, a layer of oxidized cellulose ('Surgicel') placed over the bleeding surface and covered with wet cotton-wool is a very effective haemostatic manoeuvre.

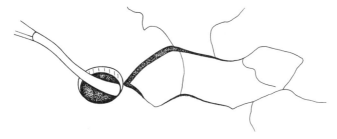

Fig. 9.3 Burr hole and elevation of fracture.

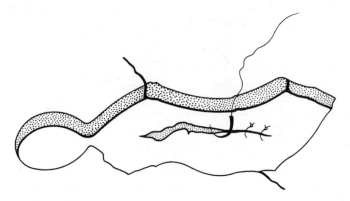

Fig. 9.4   Dural laceration repair.

If the skull defect is small (diameter: 2–3 cm) the bone fragments may be discarded, unless this will produce a cosmetic blemish—which might be the case, for example, if the fracture were below the hairline in the frontal area.

In larger defects the bone fragments are replaced. They may simply lie comfortably in place once the pericranium has been sutured; but larger fractures may have to be fixed with wire. Repair the wound in two layers using a 2/0 absorbable material to suture the galea and interrupted non-absorbable material for the skin.

Prophylactic antibiotics should be prescribed (see p. 92).

Procedures for extradural haematoma

A burr hole alone is of no value at all in the management of a solid extradural haematoma. Two procedures are described here for the treatment of this condition; but the ideal is to carry out a craniotomy.

The site of the haematoma is determined by the computerized tomo-graphy (CT) scan, or by the clinical signs if a scan is not available or clinical urgency precludes any further delay. The intracranial haematoma will cause a contralateral hemiparesis and dilatation of the ipsilateral pupil. The extradural haematoma is usually closely related to the site of the fracture, and the skull opening should be centred on the fracture site.

The proposed incision should be marked on the skin, and the scalp should be shaved. The head must be supported on a head ring. In order to prevent rotation of the neck the patient may have to be half rolled to one side and supported by sandbags. Rotation of the neck causes obstruction of cerebral venous return, and exacerbates intracranial hypertension.

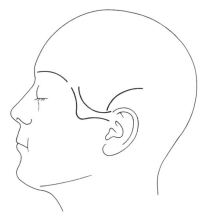

Fig. 9.5 Scalp incision.

Burr hole and craniectomy

Infiltration of the scalp with 1% lignocaine and adrenaline 1/200 000 reduces scalp bleeding.

A 7–8 cm vertical scalp incision (Fig. 9.5) is made within the hairline, and self-retaining retractors are inserted. The pericranium and temporal fascia are incised in the same line as the wound, and a periosteal elevator is used to separate the muscle from the skull. The self-retaining retractors are then replaced in this deeper plane, and the muscle is retracted. The fracture should now be evident.

A burr hole is now fashioned, first using the perforator and then the burr attached to the brace and bit. The burr hole is placed adjacent to the fracture, and care must be taken lest the bit should slip through the fracture.

Having completed the burr hole, the diagnosis will be confirmed by the sight of black haematoma extruding from the extradural space. Bright red blood is due to fresh bleeding caused by surgery, and does *not* represent haematoma! The bone defect must now be extended using a bone rongeur to enlarge the burr hole until the margins of the haematoma are seen. Bleeding from the bone is controlled by bone wax smeared into the skull margin.

The bulk of the haematoma can now be removed by suction or with forceps; but it is advisable to leave a thin layer of haematoma adherent to the dura, since this is providing haemostasis. (See Fig. 9.6.)

The dura should now be covered with a large piece of wet cotton-wool, which, if left for 5–10 minutes, will stop most of the haemorrhage from the dural surface. The cotton-wool is then washed off with saline. A

(a) (b)

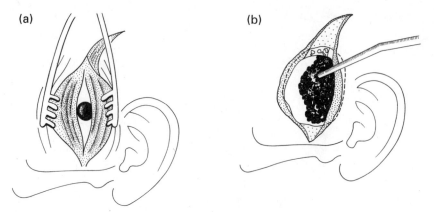

Fig. 9.6   Burr hole extended to allow craniectomy.

few bleeding points may then be seen to persist, and these can be coagulated with monopolar diathermy or covered with oxidized cellulose.

Bleeding from under the bone edges can be controlled by suturing the
dura to the pericranium at intervals.

Once absolute haemostasis has been achieved the pericranium and
temporalis muscles are sutured. A suction drain is inserted in the subgaleal layer, and the wound is closed in two layers with 2/0 absorbable
sutures to the galea and interrupted non-absorbable sutures to the skin
(Fig. 9.7).

The disadvantage of this procedure is that the skull defect will have to
be repaired at a later date using artificial material. It does, however, have
the attraction of simplicity.

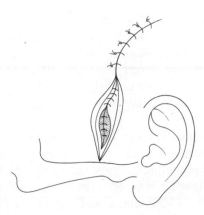

Fig. 9.7   Closure of the wound.

Craniotomy

Depending on the site of the fracture, the scalp incision is planned in order to place the wound inside the hairline and to ensure that the scalp flap retains an adequate blood supply. Mark the proposed skin incision with an indelible pen (see Fig. 9.8).

Prepare and drape the scalp, and then infiltrate the course of the proposed scalp incision with 1% lignocaine and adrenaline 1/200 000.

The surgeon and assistant compress the scalp against the skull by fingertip pressure while the incision is made in stages. At each stage, the galea is picked up with artery forceps and everted. The handles of the forceps are grouped together and retained by an elastic band.

Once the incision has been completed, the scalp flap is elevated by dissection in the plane between the galea and the pericranium or temporalis fascia. The skin flap is then wrapped in a wet swab and turned

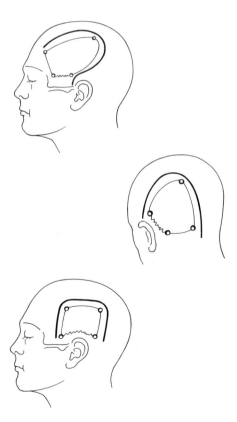

Fig. 9.8 Examples of scalp incisions.

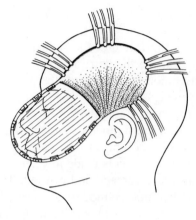

Fig. 9.9   Fashioning the wound.

down on its base to expose the pericranium and temporalis fascia. Bleeding from the skin edges is arrested by diathermy coagulation.

The pericranium and temporalis muscle are incised using cutting diathermy, following the margin of the skin incision but leaving a broad pedicle at the inferior edge on which the bone flap will be reflected (Fig. 9.9).

The pericranium is scraped back with the periosteal elevator, but should be left attached to the centre of the bone flap. Self-retaining retractors are used to spread the incision in the muscle on either side of the muscle pedicle.

At this stage the fracture should be evident. Burr holes are fashioned at the four corners of the proposed bone flap using the Hudson brace and perforator, followed by the burr (Fig. 9.10). Black clot may issue from

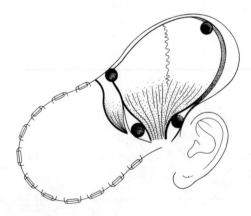

Fig. 9.10   Incision in the pericranium.

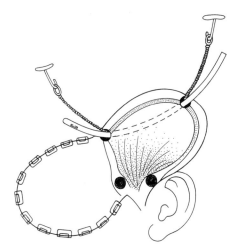

Fig. 9.11 Fashioning the craniotomy.

the burr holes, confirming the diagnosis. A blunt dissector (Adson's) is used to separate the dura gently from the skull at each burr hole.

The saw guide is passed in the plane between the skull and the dura from one burr hole to the next, and the Gigli saw is threaded between the two holes. The saw handles are attached, and, by a steady to-and-fro action, the skull is sawed between the burr holes. This is repeated at three sides of the proposed bone flap, while the anterior margin is left intact.

A periosteal elevator is then inserted through the bone incision, and the bone flap is levered up until the remaining edge of the flap fractures, allowing the bone flap to be turned back (Fig. 9.11). The bone edges may bleed, and this is controlled by pressing bone wax into the cut edge of the bone.

The bone flap now remains attached to the skull by temporalis muscle and pericranium. It is wrapped in a wet swab, and reflected with the skin flap.

The extradural haematoma is now exposed as a mass of solid clot (Fig. 9.12). The clot is removed by suction; but it is a good idea to leave a thin layer of haematoma on the dura in order to avoid provoking further dural bleeding. The dura should be covered with a large piece of wet cotton-wool which is left undisturbed for 10 minutes. This allows diffuse oozing from the dural surface to settle, and leaves the main sources of bleeding to be dealt with. The cotton-wool is then lifted off as the dura is irrigated with saline. Irrigation prevents the clot being avulsed from small bleeding points.

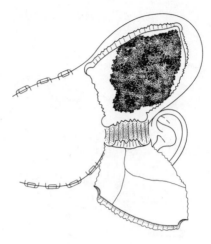

Fig. 9.12   Elevation of a bone flap.

Attention can now be turned to the main sources of haemorrhage. A common source is the middle meningeal artery, where it is severed in the fracture. Bleeding from the artery is controlled by coagulation with monopolar diathermy. If the artery is injured in the skull base the bleeding is easily controlled by pressing bone wax into the fracture or the foramen spinosum. This is much easier than using the sterile matchstick referred to in some textbooks, and is usually more readily available! Other bleeding points on the dura can be coagulated or covered with haemostatic gauze (oxidized cellulose or Surgicel). (See Fig. 9.13.)

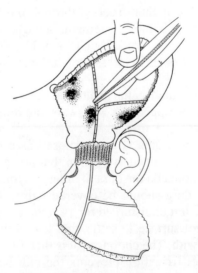

Fig. 9.13   Coagulation of the middle meningeal artery.

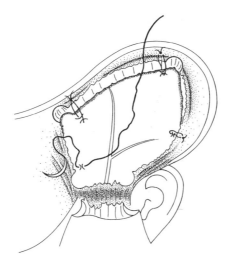

Fig. 9.14 Hitching the dura.

Frequently, dural bleeding is found to be a diffuse ooze, and not to arise from a single meningeal vessel.

Bleeding from the extradural space under the edges of the craniotomy can be troublesome, and is controlled by sliding a piece of haemostatic gauze between the bone and the dura. If bleeding is heavy the dura can be hitched up to the skull by suturing it to the pericranium (Fig. 9.14).

Once **all** bleeding has ceased the bone flap is replaced and held in position by suturing the pericranium with interrupted 2/0 absorbable sutures.

A suction drain is placed between the pericranium and the skin flap, and the flap is replaced. The skin flap is sutured in two layers. Interrupted 2/0 sutures are used to approximate the edges of the galea, and the skin is closed with interrupted nylon or silk (Fig. 9.15).

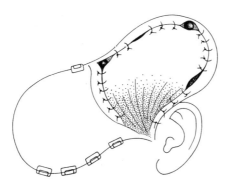

Fig. 9.15 Suture of the pericranium.

The head is bandaged. The drain is removed after 24 hours, and skin sutures are removed after 3 days.

When no extradural haematoma is found

Even when CT scanning facilities are available misinterpretation of the scan may lead to an erroneous diagnosis of extradural haematoma when the lesion is really subdural or intracerebral. In these circumstances no extradural haematoma is found, but the dura is tense and bulging. This creates considerable difficulty for the inexperienced surgeon, who must then decide whether to proceed to open the dura or whether to abandon the procedure and seek neurosurgical help. If the latter is not practical the dura should be incised and opened in a cruciate fashion. Obvious subdural haematoma may then be removed by a combination of suction and irrigation with normal saline. It should be remembered that the subdural haematoma is usually associated with severe primary brain injury, and the underlying brain will be swollen. Unless the dura is closed rapidly the brain will tend to herniate through the craniotomy, and the wound will become progressively more difficult to close.

If surgery is thought to be necessary in the base hospital it is more likely that no CT scan is available to guide the procedure. If no extradural haematoma is found this may be due to incorrect location of the craniotomy, or to the fact that the haematoma is intradural. The craniotomy may be incorrectly sited if the haematoma is situated very anteriorly or posteriorly, or when the site of the skull fracture has been misinterpreted. In these circumstances the dura should be cautiously incised to identify a subdural haematoma, and if this is absent the wound should be closed (Fig. 9.16) and the patient should be transferred as soon as is practical to a specialist centre.

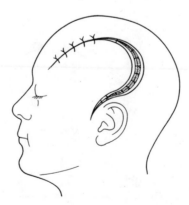

Fig. 9.16   Closure of the scalp wound.

Further reading

Gudeman, S. K. (1989). Indications for operative treatment and operative technique in closed head injuries. In *Textbook of head injury* (ed. D. P. Becker and S. K. Gudeman), pp. 182–191. W. B. Saunders, Philadelphia.

Keenan, R. *et al.* (1989). Surgical anaesthesia in head injury. In *Textbook of head injury* (ed. D. P. Becker and S. K. Gudeman), pp. 182–91. W. B. Saunders, Philadelphia.

Symon, I., Thomas, D. G., and Clark, K. (ed) (1989). Rob and Smith's *operative surgery, Neurosurgery* (4th edn). Butterworth, London.

10 Anaesthesia in head injuries

Chapter contents

Key points in anaesthesia for head injuries

1 An experienced Anaesthetist is an essential part of the team responsible for resuscitation and transfer of the head injured patient.
2 Raised $PaCO_2$ and low PaO_2 cause increased intracranial pressure.
3 Monitoring of physiological parameters and correction of hypovolaemia, hypoxia, and hypercapnia must be established before surgery or transportation.
4 Anaesthetic technique should aim to control intracranial pressure and preserve cerebral perfusion.
5 Anaesthetic technique and choice of drugs can adversely affect intracranial pressure and cerebral perfusion.
6 The head-injured patient is at risk of aspiration of gastric contents.
7 Postoperative ventilation should be considered if the preoperative Glasgow Coma Score was less than 8, if there were uncontrolled fits, if there is any risk of respiratory insufficiency, if there are multiple injuries, or if raised intracranial pressure is anticipated.
8 Antiemetic drugs should be used prophylactically to reduce the risk of vomiting and aspiration of gastric contents after extubation.

The anaesthetist is a key member of the team involved in the care of the head-injured patient. The anaesthetist is involved in the transfer of head-injured patients both within the hospital and between hospitals, in the resuscitation of the patient and in anaesthesia for surgical procedures. A thorough understanding of the pathology, physiology, and pharmacology of anaesthetic drugs is required for the safe conduct of these tasks.

An estimated 50% of severely head-injured patients who are admitted to hospital die and only 25% make a recovery without lasting disability. Thirty per cent of this group have other injuries, 8% severe, and 51% experience airway difficulty; 21% have associated chest trauma. In the light of such unfavourable statistics, it is clear that skilled resuscitation and subsequent anaesthetic attention plays a vital part in protecting the patient from death and serious disability. Anaesthesia for head-injured patients should, therefore, be carried out by experienced anaesthetists. Inexpert anaesthetic technique can certainly contribute to secondary brain injury.

Physiology

As previously described, secondary brain injury can be caused by reduced cerebral perfusion, hypoxia, anaemia, and endogenous mediator release. The goal for the anaesthetist is to minimize or ameliorate secondary cerebral insults. Initial hypotension in the head-injured patient carries a 50% increase in mortality. Providing well-oxygenated blood containing glucose at a sufficient rate to the brain tissue is paramount to nerve cell survival.

The relationship between brain volume (and hence intracranial pressure) and systemic arterial pressure, central venous pressure, and arterial carbon dioxide tension ($PaCO_2$) has been described in Chapter 1. Their relationships to cerebral blood flow are demonstrated in Fig. 10.1. The physiology of intracranial pressure, cerebral blood flow, and cerebrovascular autoregulation is central to the management of anaesthesia in head-injured patients and is discussed in greater detail here.

The volume of the contents of the cranium includes the volume of brain tissue, cerebrospinal fluid, and cerebral blood vessels. The calibre

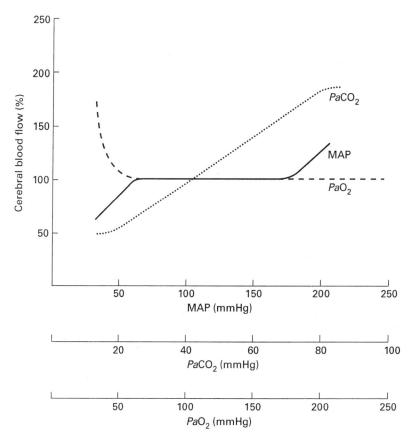

Fig. 10.1 The relationship of mean arterial pressure (MAP), $PaCO_2$, and PaO_2 to cerebral blood flow.

of the blood vessels is the main parameter that can be manipulated by the anaesthetist in order to control intracranial pressure (ICP) and, hence, cerebral perfusion. The intracranial blood volume is altered by systemic arterial pressure, central venous pressure, and the calibre of the cerebral arterioles. The latter is principally affected by arterial carbon dioxide tension ($PaCO_2$) and arterial oxygen tension (PaO_2), (see Fig. 10.1). A rise in $PaCO_2$ causes cerebral arteriolar dilatation and an increase in ICP. A decrease in PaO_2 can produce a sixfold increase in cerebral blood flow. Decreasing $PaCO_2$, on the other hand, can bring about a reduction in intracranial pressure—hence the use of hyperventilation to regulate ICP in severely head-injured patients. Conversely, reduction of $PaCO_2$ below 3 kPa may cause cerebral ischaemia due to excessive vasoconstriction. Damaged areas of brain may be relatively immune to this effect, however, since there is a local vasodilatation which is unresponsive to lowering of $PaCO_2$. The effects of raised $PaCO_2$ and reduced PaO_2 are additive.

The cranium and dura can be regarded as a rigid box. If there is an expansion in the contents, due to haematoma or brain swelling, the intracranial pressure will be elevated. Initially, there is a minimal increase in ICP due to a compensatory displacement of intravascular blood and cerebrospinal fluid (CSF), (see Fig. 10.2). Once a critical increase in volume has been reached and compensation fails, a relatively small further increase in volume will produce a relatively large increase in ICP with a concomitant reduction in cerebral perfusion. The critical factor in these processes is the effect on cerebral perfusion. Cerebral blood flow (CBF) is determined by the cerebral perfusion pressure (CPP) and the cerebrovascu-

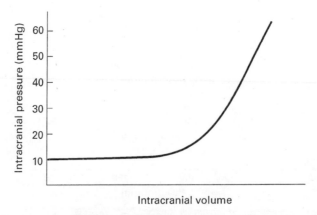

Fig. 10.2   The relationship between intracranial volume and intracranial pressure.

Box 10.1   Causes of increased cerebral blood flow (CBF)

- Increased $PaCO_2$
- Decreased PaO_2
- Impaired autoregulation
- Increased MAP

lar resistance (Box 10.1). The CPP is determined by the mean systemic arterial pressure (MAP) and the ICP according to the formula:

$$CPP = MAP - ICP.$$

It is known that, in head-injured patients, the normal autoregulatory mechanism of CBF is damaged and this effect may last for as much as 5 days after injury. A fall in MAP is not compensated for by a corresponding increase in CBF with the result that, in the presence of constant or rising ICP, there is a reduction in cerebral perfusion. If cerebral perfusion falls below a critical level anaerobic metabolism will occur and this will ultimately lead to irreversible cell damage. On the other hand, an excessive rise in MAP will result in increased CBF and increased cerebral blood volume, resulting in an increase in ICP.

A rise in central venous pressure will lead to a reduction in cerebral venous drainage and an increase intracranial blood volume, also causing a rise in ICP. Reduction in cerebral venous return may be caused by the following factors; rotation of the neck, tilting the patient head-down, applying collars or tapes to the neck, allowing the patient to cough or 'fight the ventilator' because of inadequate sedation or paralysis, and causes of raised intrathoracic pressure such as pneumothorax (Box 10.2).

Box 10.2   Causes of reduced cerebral venous return

- Neck rotation
- Head-down tilt
- Collars applied directly to neck
- Tapes tied round neck
- Coughing against resistance
- Raised intrathoracic pressure

Box 10.3   Techniques for lowering intracranial pressure (ICP)

- Hyperventilation
- Adequate oxygenation
- Head-up tilt
- Prevention of neck rotation
- Avoid tapes round neck
- Prevent coughing/spontaneous respiration
- Diuretics/osmotic agents (e.g. mannitol)

The brain can only survive complete cessation of perfusion, oxygenation, and the supply of glucose substrate at normothermia for 3–4 minutes. This is due to its low energy stores and high metabolic requirement for oxygen ($CMRO_2$). The critical level of CPP is about 50 mmHg. Between 40 and 25 mmHg the EEG decreases in frequency and amplitude. Below 20 mmHg, cell wall integrity fails and irreversible damage occurs.

Employing the physiology described above, the anaesthetist is able to regulate ICP and cerebral perfusion during resuscitation and in the operating theatre in order to prevent secondary brain injury (Box 10.3).

Pharmacology

Anaesthetic agents can alter the physiological responses in head-injured patients and can be used to provide a degree of neuronal protection by reducing $CMRO_2$. Anaesthetic drugs and techniques can, on the other hand, contribute to rises in ICP and cause unwanted reductions in MAP. The possible contribution of drugs to raised ICP is of less concern in the operating theatre when the skull has been opened than it is in resuscitation or during ventilation in the intensive care unit.

Induction agents

Thiopentone, propofol, and **etomidate** are used as induction agents in head-injured patients. **Thiopentone** reduces $CMRO_2$ and ICP by causing cerebral vasoconstriction. In addition, it has anticonvulsant properties. Its theoretical benefits as a neuroprotective agent tend to be cancelled out by undesirable cardiovascular effects and it is not now routinely used in the intensive care of head-injured patients. In the hypovolaemic patient, its hypotensive effects are exaggerated and it must be used with caution. **Propofol** has similar properties to thiopentone and has the theoretical benefit of being a free radical scavenger. It may be used as an infusion intraoperatively and in the intensive care unit postoperatively. Again, it should be used with caution in the hypovolaemic patient. **Etomidate** has similar properties to thiopentone with the added advantage of providing greater cardiovascular stability, cell membrane stabilization, and attenuation of free fatty acid liberation. It does, however, tend to cause nausea and vomiting which are undesirable in the postoperative head-injured patient. It should not be used as an infusion because of possible adrenocortical suppression. **Ketamine** causes an increase in cerebral oxygen consumption ($CMRO_2$) and ICP and should be avoided.

Opioids

To obtund the stress response and surge in blood pressure seen at intubation and to prevent intraoperative hypertension an opioid is desirable. Short-acting opioids are essential in order to avoid long-lasting effects and to aid early neurological assessment of the patient on reversal of anaesthesia. **Fentanyl** is the opioid of choice, having minimal effects on $CMRO_2$ and cerebral haemodynamics. **Alfentanyl** and **sufentanyl** produce a significant decrease in cerebral perfusion pressure (CPP) in bolus form due to a decrease in mean arterial pressure (MAP) and a rise in ICP. This does not occur when **alfentanyl** is used as an infusion. **Remifentanyl** as an infusion does not raise ICP and has the added benefit over **fentanyl** of decreasing time to awakening. Although remifentanyl has only recently become available it may become the agent of choice.

Muscle relaxants

The head-injured patient may require rapid muscle paralysis. There is theoretical risk that the initial muscle contraction caused by **suxamethonium** might bring about a rise in ICP but this has been observed only in conjunction with laryngoscopy, and the benefits of rapid intubation justify its use. **Rocuronium** is almost as rapidly acting as suxamethonium but its longer action may be undesirable if intubation fails. If rapid control of the airway is not essential, **vecuronium** and **atracurium** cause no change in ICP or $CMRO_2$. Atracurium is metabolized to laudanosine which, if it accumulates, can cause convulsions. **Pancuronium** should be avoided as it has the effect of increasing systemic blood pressure, cerebral blood flow, and intracranial pressure.

Maintenance anaesthetic agents

All volatile anaesthetic agents cause cerebral vasodilatation in proportion to their partial pressure, but **isoflurane** is the least inclined to do so and is the most effective in reducing $CMRO_2$. Of the volatile anaesthetic agents, therefore, isoflurane is the most appropriate in head-injury anaesthesia. Prior hyperventilation may reduce the vasodilator effect of all the volatile agents but this may not be sufficient to prevent a rise in ICP in severe head injury. the combination of **thiopentone**, with its vasoconstrictor effect, used with small concentrations of a volatile agent, and hyperventilation provides anaesthesia with control of intracranial pressure.

Perioperative management

The anaesthetist's involvement with the head-injured patient commonly begins at the stage of resuscitation and the patient remains in the care of the anaesthetist during transfer within the hospital or between hospitals, in the operating theatre, and in the intensive care unit. Under the anaesthetist's care, the patient may have to be moved within the hospital to X-ray departments, in lifts, along corridors or, indeed, between hospitals. Attention to detail in preparation and monitoring is of the utmost importance.

Other injuries frequently complicate anaesthetic management and pre-anaesthetic assessment is important. The time available for assessment depends on the urgency of resuscitation and surgery. Intubation may be complicated by facial lacerations and swelling, by injuries of the facial skeleton, and by the presence of cervical spine injuries. The anaesthetist should be aware of the presence of chest injury and a history of aspiration of gastric contents. The patient with significant pulmonary complications will require continuing ventilation until respiratory function has improved.

Correction of hypovolaemia is essential in order to maintain cerebral perfusion and prior to anaesthesia since anaesthesia agents may cause further hypotension. Hypovolaemia may be due to blood loss from other injuries or to diuresis following the administration of diuretic agents and further loss of blood volume should be anticipated if an operation is to follow.

Early investigations of importance include a chest X-ray, arterial blood gas analysis, haemoglobin, and serum electrolytes. Blood should be cross-matched for transfusion before proceeding to surgery.

A skilled anaesthetic assistant should be available, along with a full range of equipment and drugs for resuscitation. Particular attention should be paid to equipment needed in the event of a difficult intubation. Electrocardiogram (ECG) monitoring and the monitoring of blood pressure and oxygen saturation should be established, and a large-bore venous cannula inserted. In the operating theatre, the following monitoring facilities will be required: inspired oxygen concentration, non-invasive blood pressure monitoring, temperature, muscle relaxation monitoring, a ventilation failure alarm, and end-tidal carbon dioxide monitoring. Direct arterial blood pressure monitoring is preferable since it may be valuable in the event of large blood losses and because it provides ready access to arterial blood samples for blood gas analysis, haemoglobin, and clotting studies. Central venous pressure monitoring is usually not required unless there are other serious injuries or when heavy blood loss is anticipated.

Induction of anaesthesia and intubation

The mode of induction of anaesthesia is based on the assumption that the patient is at risk of aspiration of gastric contents and on the predicted ease of intubation. After trauma, it can be assumed that the stomach remains full for 24–48 hours and a rapid sequence induction is usually necessary. A nasogastric tube should not be passed preoperatively s this will lead to coughing and retching and an increase in intracranial pressure.

The choice of induction agent depends on personal preference. **Thiopentone**, **propofol**, and **etomidate** are all satisfactory. An opioid to obtund the stress response is desirable. The author's preference is for **fentanyl** (2–4 mcg/kg). **Lignocaine** and **beta-blockers** have been used for the same purpose.

Since the stomach is assumed to be full, rapid intubation conditions are required and this can be achieved using **suxamethonium** as a paralysing agent. Thereafter, neuromuscular monitoring is essential in order to detect loss of muscle relaxation which will lead to the patient coughing on the endotracheal tube. If possible, it is also helpful to have neuromuscular monitoring at the time of induction in order to be able to be sure that full muscle relaxation has occurred before intubation. This is particularly desirable when using long-acting muscle relaxants. Neuromuscular monitoring is also essential to assess the degree of recovery from muscle relaxants before extubation.

During intubation, there should be as little traction on the larynx as possible in order to avoid surges in blood pressures and intracranial pressure. Before laryngoscopy, a further bolus of intravenous induction agent will help to obtund this response. A reinforced endotracheal tube should be used in order to avoid kinking if the patient's head is turned to one side. An assistant should maintain pressure on the cricoid during laryngoscopy to prevent regurgitation of gastric contents. Careful attention should be paid to the positioning of the endotracheal tube which, owing to its uncut length, is more likely to migrate down the right main bronchus. The endotracheal tube should be secured with tape to the face in order to avoid compression of the neck veins which may occur if it is tied in place with tapes. The eyes should be protected and a throat pack used to prevent a leak should the endotracheal cuff burst during surgery.

Insertion of a urinary catheter should be considered if a long surgical procedure is anticipated. If **mannitol** has to be used a catheter enables the anaesthetist to calculate intravenous fluid requirements and helps to prevent postoperative discomfort. A nasogastric tube should be passed in order to empty the stomach and for the purpose of initiating feeding as soon as possible in the postoperative period when very high catabolism creates serious nutritional demands. If there is a coexisting fracture of the anterior skull base an orogastric tube should be used instead.

When the patient is being positioned for surgery, great care must be taken to prevent displacement of the endotracheal tube. All pressure areas should be padded and good drainage of the neck veins ensured. If head stabilization devices using pins are to be used a small bolus narcotic or intravenous induction agent may be required to obtund any pressor response. The operating table should be tilted head-up if cardiovascular stability permits. At this point, hypotension should be anticipated and treated, if necessary, with pressor drugs or intravenous fluids. A head-up tilt of up to 30° leads to a reduction in blood pressure and intracranial pressure, but no change in cerebral perfusion pressure, cerebral blood flow, or $CMRO_2$.

Intraoperative management

Maintenance of anaesthesia can be continued with either a volatile agent, total intravenous anaesthesia or, more rarely, with neuroleptic anaesthesia. Conventionally, the volatile agent of choice is isoflurane since it causes minimal cerebral vasodilatation. Surgical stimulus is maximal at incision of the skin, raising the craniotomy bone flap and during skin closure. A bolus of opioid or propofol will obtund the effects of these stimuli.

During anaesthesia and surgery the following physiological parameters should be regulated: **body temperature** should be monitored and both hypothermia and hyperthermia avoided; a PaO_2 of about 15 kPa is desirable in order to prevent vasodilatation and preserve good oxygenation. If adequate oxygenation is difficult to achieve the cause should be identified and treated. The introduction of positive end-expiratory pressure (PEEP) up to 15 cmH$_2$O in a patient with raised intracranial pressure (ICP) does not cause a further rise in ICP. In the absence of raised ICP, PEEP of greater than 5 cmH$_2$O will cause a rise in ICP but no reduction in cerebral perfusion pressure (CPP). A $PaCO_2$ of about 4 kPa provides vasoconstriction, a reduction in ICP, and improved surgical conditions but does not impair cerebral perfusion. The mean arterial pressure (MAP) should be maintained above 80 mmHg and the systolic blood pressure above 110 mmHg while avoiding hypertension.

There is controversy over the choice of crystalloids or colloids for intravenous fluid replacement. However, it is now established that, although hypoglycaemia may be catastrophic for the injured brain, hyperglycaemia may also exacerbate neurological damage. In the absence of hypoglycaemia, dextrose-containing solutions should be avoided. Increased capillary permeability in head injury allows extravasation of colloid into the extravascular space, drawing water into the brain tissue. It seems logical to use non-dextrose-containing crystalloids (0.9% salline or Hartmann's solution) for the maintenance of fluid balance and reserve colloids and blood for volume expansion.

Postoperative care

It is necessary, at the end of the surgical procedure, to decide whether there are advantages in continuing to ventilate the patient (Box 10.4). Early extubation is desirable unless there are good indications or continuing to ventilate the patient. Prolonged ventilation is not free from

Box 10.4   Indications for postoperative ventilation

- Preoperative Glasgow Coma Score < 8
- Inability to protect/maintain adequate airway
- Uncontrolled convulsions preoperatively
- Preoperative hyperventilation : $PaCO_2$ < 3 kPa
- Preoperative hypoventilation : PaO_2 < 6 kPa
- Multiple injuries especially thoracic
- PaO_2 < 10 kPa on supplemental oxygen
- Anticipated continuing raised ICP

hazards—principally of chest infection and the acquisition of resistant infections in the intensive care unit. Any suggestion, however, that there may be respiratory difficulties in the immediate postoperative period should be an absolute indication for ventilation. Thus, patients who had respiratory difficulties prior to surgery and those with significant chest or lung injuries should be ventilated. Patients with facial injuries may be unable to maintain a patent upper airway if consciousness is impaired. It may be clear from the computerized tomography (CT) scan and from the findings at operation, that further swelling of the brain can be expected after resuscitation or operation. Thus continuing ventilation may be required specifically to control intracranial pressure (ICP). In these circumstances it is ideal to use ICP monitoring to enable rational decisions to be made about the duration of ventilation and the patient's physiological management. Areas of cerebral contusion can swell and do, on occasion, require surgical intervention. If a CT scan has been carried out very early it is possible for intracranial haematomas to develop after scanning. In both these circumstances ICP monitoring allows recognition of the increasing intracranial mass.

If there have been frequent fits prior to ventilation or if there has been an episode of status epilepticus, postoperative ventilation allows a period of stability during which anticonvulsant medication can be established (Box 10.5).

If extubation is intended, antiemetic drugs should be given to minimize postoperative retching or vomiting. The 5HT-3 antagonists such as **domperidone** or **ondansetron** have the advantage of causing minimal sedation.

It is undesirable to allow the patient to cough or gag on the endotracheal tube for a prolonged period of time before extubation. On the other hand, the patient must be breathing effectively and protecting the upper airway once the tube is removed.

Box 10.5   Drugs used for postoperative ventilation

Drug	Bolus dose	Infusion rate
Propofol	2.5–5 mg	0.5–6 mg/h
Midazolam	1–2.5 mg/kg	1–4 mg/h
Fentanyl	25–100 ug	100–200 ug/h
Alfentanyl	250 ug	1–6 mg/h
Atracurium	300–600 ug/kg	300–600 mcg/kg/h
Vecuronium	40–100 ug/kg	40–80 mcg/kg/h

After extubation, the adequacy of respiration should be confirmed clinically and, if necessary, by arterial blood gas analysis. Supplemental oxygen should be supplied and the patient should be nursed in a high-dependency area where close neurological monitoring is possible. Postoperative analgesia should avoid sedation and should not affect the reactions of the pupils. **Codeine phosphate** combined, if necessary, with **paracetamol** often provides adequate analgesia. In the fully conscious patient with other painful injuries, however, a more powerful opioid analgesic may be indicated. However, non-steroidal antiinflamatory drugs should be avoided because of the high incidence of upper gastrointestinal haemorrhage in head-injured patients.

Further reading

Michenfield, J. D. (1990). *Anaesthesia and the brain*. Churchill Livingstone, New York.

Hinds, J. C. and Watson, D. (1996). *Head injuries and raised intracranial pressure in intensive care: A concise textbook*, (2nd edn). W. B. Saunders, Philadelphia.

11 *The disturbed head-injured patient*

Chapter contents

Key points in managing disturbed head-injured patients

1   Disturbed behaviour may be due to a medical condition that caused the head injury.
2   Drunkenness cannot be assumed to be the cause of abnormal behaviour in the head-injured patient.
3   Disordered behaviour may be due to a medical condition coexisting with the head injury.
4   The restless patient should not be sedated.
5   Extreme restlessness may be due to hypoxia, urinary retention hypoglycaemia, drug overdose, or intracranial haematoma.
6   When aggressive and uncooperative behaviour may be due to head injury the patient may require forcible restraint in order to exclude an intracranial haematoma.
7   Decisions about the management of the disruptive head-injured patient require the presence of experienced senior medical staff.

Managing the disturbed head injured patient

Disturbed behaviour is common after head injuries when there is some degree of altered consciousness. Inspection of the Glasgow Coma Scale (See Box 1.3) will show that a minor degree of altered consciousness results in 'confusion' even although the patient remains ambulant and able to obey commands. A further deterioration in consciousness results in a verbal response described as 'inappropriate words'. This commonly means that the patient is abusive and uses offensive language. This is usually a transient phenomenon requiring little active intervention but it is of the greatest importance that those responsible for dealing with head-injured patients realize that this behaviour indicates altered consciousness and not simply antisocial behaviour or drunkenness.

Serious behavioural disturbance may, in its own right, pose problems in the management of the patient as well as indicating that there has been some form of cerebral insult. It may be a danger to the patient, to other patients, and members of hospital staff. This problem calls for a high degree of professionalism from doctors and nurses in the face of abuse, aggression, and uncooperative behaviour. However, disturbing and disorderly behaviour must be regarded as a part of the head-injured patient's symptomatology and not simply as antisocial behaviour.

Disorderly behaviour after head injury includes the irritable state commonly seen in partially conscious patients—the extreme form of restlessness with hectic purposeless thrashing around seen after head injuries and, especially, anoxic brain injury. In addition, uncooperative, violent behaviour is seen in some head-injured patients who remain ambulant and able to express their refusal to accept treatment. These patients may be impossible to distinguish from the plain drunk and disorderly. A variety of other medical conditions can also present with behavioural disorders and these must be considered even when there is a history of head injury and especially when there is no clear history from witnesses. Failure to recognize that disturbed behaviour is due to a medical condition and, in particular, to a complication of a head injury can and does result in delayed treatment or even the death of the patient. In an A&E department that has to deal with drunken citizens who may have had an injury or may simply be drunk and disorderly, heavy demands are placed on staff who may have to devote a disproportionate amount of time to the disruptive drunk at the expense of other patients. The law, however, deals harshly with the professionals who miss the medical condition in these circumstances and an awareness of this problem is important for the protection of the doctor or nurse as well as for the patient.

Causes for disturbed behaviour

The head-injured patient may have other medical conditions that contributed to the accident. One of the requirements in the assessment of the head-injured patient is to establish, in the history from the patient and witnesses, whether the injury might have been caused by some preceding illness or the consumption of prescribed or illicit drugs. The same condition may cause continuing symptoms after admission to hospital with a head injury.

Medical conditions

A very large number of medical conditions can present with delirium and the more common ones are listed in Box 11.1.

It is important to check the blood glucose level in all head-injured patients with altered consciousness or disturbed behaviour. Initially, use a glucose stick test and treat hypoglycaemia immediately, but if the stick test registers low blood glucose, confirm the result by taking blood for a formal blood glucose analysis.

Evidence of drug abuse should be sought and a history of prescribed drugs obtained as soon as possible. The injuries may have been caused by disturbed behaviour or attempted suicide in patients with psychotic

Box 11.1   Common causes of disturbed behaviour

Metabolic	– Hypoglycaemia
Poisoning	– Sympathomimetics
Drug Abuse	– Ecstasy
	– LSD
Alcohol	– Intoxication
	– Withdrawal
Hypoxia	
Infection	
Psychiatric conditions	– Psychoses
	– Manipulative patients
	– Munchausen's syndrome
Epilepsy	– Complex partial seizures

conditions and psychotic behavioural disturbance is sometimes seen as a response to injury, particularly assault. Alcohol intoxication is a common factor in the aetiology of head injury but alcohol withdrawal symptoms may also result in injury and continuing behavioural disturbance. Epilepsy is a very rare cause of bizarre behaviour but should be remembered as an occasional cause of paroxysmal abnormal behaviour in patients who have had head injuries.

Complications of the head injury

Post-concussional irritability

Following a concussional head injury and while the conscious level remains depressed, the patient is commonly irritable, resenting examination, recordings, and attempts to treat lacerations or apply dressings. Left undisturbed, such patients will often curl up and sleep between observations. Attempts at examination are often met by abuse and resistance. The patient may pull out intravenous lines and monitoring equipment. This behaviour resolves as the conscious level improves. It is usually futile to try to gain the patient's cooperation during this phase. It is reasonable to delay procedures, such as suturing lacerations, rather than resorting to restraint or general anaesthesia. The nurse has to be vigilant in case the patient tries to get out of bed and cot sides are useful to prevent the patient suffering further injuries in hospital.

> **Sedation is strictly to be avoided**

The restless patient may fail to lie sufficiently still to allow skull X-rays or a computerized tomography (CT) scan to be carried out. It may be necessary to anaesthetize the patient in order to do so. But it should be remembered that there are hazards in anaesthetizing an injured patient who may have a full stomach and other, as yet unrecognized, injuries. An alternative policy is to admit the patient for observation in a unit where skilled neurological observation can be carried out by nurses who are familiar with neurological observation and, preferably, under the care of a neurosurgeon. If this policy is adopted the patient may be seen to be improving spontaneously and investigation can continue to be deferred. If, on the other hand, deterioration is observed and the patient remains too restless to be scanned it will be necessary to proceed to a general anaesthetic and a CT scan. At the time of admission, the patient may have been drowsy and prepared to curl up and sleep when undisturbed. Disturbed, restless behaviour developing after an initial period of drowsiness should not be interpreted as an improvement in consciousness. It is an ominous sign of cerebral disturbance indicating a delayed complication of the head injury such as an intracranial haematoma.

Extreme restlessness in the unconscious patient

Hectic restless behaviour in the head-injured patient may be both a feature of the injury and an obstacle to assessment. It may be a feature of the primary brain injury, particularly when this has been associated with hypoxia. Continuing hypoxia due to chest injury may cause severe restlessness. The patient may, for example, have a pneumothorax or upper airway obstruction. When this behaviour develops after a delay, during which the patient has been quiet and irritable only when disturbed, it may herald a rising intracranial pressure due to an intracranial haematoma. It is also seen as a response to a full bladder in the unconscious patient. It may also be a feature of drug overdose and hypoglycaemia. (See Box 11.2.)

The patient thrashes around on the examination trolley in a puposeless fashion. There is sweating, tachycardia, and hyperventilation. It may be impossible to conduct an examination, insert an intravenous line, or carry

Box 11.2   Causes of extreme restlessness

Anoxic brain injury
Continuing hypoxia   – Chest injury
                                      – Pneumothorax
                                      – Upper airway obstruction

Hypoglycaemia
Urinary retention .
Intracranial haematoma
Drug overdose
Alcohol withdrawal

out investigations. In these circumstances, further management is often impossible without a general anaesthetic. In the case of the patient who has had an anoxic brain injury, ventilation for 24 hours may be sufficient to allow this problem to settle. A CT scan is mandatory once the patient has been anaesthetized.

The patient should never be sedated.

The ambulant disturbed patient

A particularly difficult problem is posed by the head-injured patient who is alert and ambulant and who is disruptive in the A&E Department. The patient may refuse attention and investigations and may be abusive and violent towards staff. Fortunately, this is a relatively rare occurrence since it poses difficult ethical, legal, and management problems. It is essential to realize that this behaviour may be a feature of the head injury and may reflect a primary brain injury or a developing intracranial mass. The doctor may be tempted to attribute this behaviour to alcohol or drugs. The circumstances of the accident are most important. Witnesses, such as the ambulance crew, may be able to give clear evidence that makes intoxication unlikely. The cyclist, for example, returning home from work is unlikely to be drunk.

It is a safe rule to always assume that the abnormal behaviour is due to the injury. If the patient is known to have suffered a head injury, disturbed behaviour cannot be safely attributed to alcohol intoxication. The dilemma is then to decide how to detain the patient and secure his/her cooperation with investigations when he/she has made it clear that he/she does not wish treatment. Every effort should be made to gain the patient's cooperation. It is not uncommon to see restless head-injured patients in A&E departments who resist attempts at examination, blood pressure recordings, or investigations and whose restlessness is made worse by attempts by the staff to restrain them. In these circumstances, the patient may become less disruptive if left to lie on a trolley or in bed and observed with minimal intervention. Observation should, ideally, be undertaken in a neurosurgery ward where the decision to delay further investigation can be taken by specialist staff. The neurosurgeon should not insist that a CT scan be carried out before transfer to a neurosurgical unit. There are occasions, however, when the ambulant confused patient cannot be contained so that observations or investigations can be carried out. Fortunately, this is not a common event. The doctor is faced with the following choices: to allow the patient to leave the department; to forceable restrain and anaesthetize the patient; to request the assistance of the police and have the patient detained in police custody. None of these courses of action are ideal and each carries serious risks for both the patient and the doctor. The decision must be made by a consultant. When it is known that the patient has had a head injury it is really not acceptable to allow him/her to leave hospital. Detention in a police cell may allow observation of a sort but it imposes an unfair responsibility on police officers who are not trained for the task. There are occasions, therefore, when one must consider forceable restraint. This course of action requires the presence of a consultant in the A&E department and a senior anaesthetist. There are risks to the patient who may have a full stomach and who may not have been adequately assessed. There is also a risk to the doctor who might be accused of assault. This has to be balanced against the certain risk of being accused of negligence if the patient dies of complications of a head injury.

The key to this problem is early diagnosis by CT scan so that confident decisions can be made about the patient's disposal without the anxiety that an intracranial lesion is being neglected.

Further reading

Plum, F. and Posner, J. (1991). *The diagnosis of stupor and coma.* F. A. Davis & Co., Philadelphia.

12 *Delayed complications*

Chapter contents

Key points in delayed complications of head injury

1 *Post-traumatic fits*. Anticonvulsants should be prescribed only if the patient has had a fit, and must then be continued indefinitely if the patient wishes to reduce the likelihood of recurrent fits. Phenytoin should be avoided in children because it causes gum hyperplasia, and sodium valproate in women of child-bearing age because of its teratogenicity. Phenobarbitone is more sedative than alternative drugs, and may cause hyperkinesia and behavioural disturbance in children.

2 *Meningitis*. The possibility of meningitis should be considered in patients who present with delayed symptoms weeks, months, or even years after a known head injury, especially a skull base fracture. The characteristic physical signs are fever and neck stiffness, which may be accompanied by reduced conscious level and focal neurological signs such as hemiparesis or cranial nerve palsies, and sometimes (usually later) papilloedema. Other common symptoms are progressive headache, neck pain, back pain, photophobia, and vomiting, and later, drowsiness, confusion, and diplopia.

3 Except when there is any suspicion of an intracranial mass, diagnosis should be confirmed, and the causative organism and its antibiotic sensitivity should be determined, by lumbar puncture. But when an intracranial mass may be present a computerized tomography (CT) scan should be ordered if available, or, if not, antibiotic therapy should be started *without* a lumbar puncture. (This course would apply for not fully recovered head-injury patients who might have intracranial haematomas or cerebral confusion, and for those presenting with altered consciousness and/or papilloedema.) In these cases blood and any discharges should be taken for culture before therapy starts.

4 Immediate antibiotic therapy before the causative organism is determined should cover all likely pathogens: a combination of benzylpenicillin, cefotaxime, and metronidazole can be used. Therapy should continue for at least 2 weeks in the absence of a cerebrospinal fluid (CSF) fistula, or until any fistula has been repaired, with the lumbar puncture repeated if there is any doubt of eradication, and continuing therapy if a raised cell count persists.

5 Once the patient has made a full recovery from infection the possibility of a CSF fistula must be investigated, and if one is found it must be repaired, or there will be a risk of recurrence.

6 *Aerocele*. A large aerocele causes severe headache, usually of rapid onset, which may be accompanied by alteration of consciousness and focal deficits such as hemiparesis. Characteristically, it occurs in a patient who has been recovering from head injury for some days or

weeks, producing a delayed deterioration. Diagnosis is easily made by plain brow-up skull X-rays, which show the collection of air in the anterior fossa. They often resolve spontaneously; but this indicates there is a significant fistula which needs surgical repair to avert the possibility of meningitis. Antibiotic prophylaxis should be given.

7 *Hydrocephalus.* A rare complication, usually of severe head injuries. Clinical features include headache, intellectual impairment, urinary incontinence, and gait disturbance. Diagnosis is by CT scan, which may also detect pre-existing symptomless hydrocephalus, not due to trauma.

8 *Chronic subdural haematoma.* Most common in the elderly and the alcoholic, and more likely in cases of cerebral atrophy. Patients present with headache, intellectual deterioration, focal neurological signs such as hemiparesis or dysphasia, and deteriorating consciousness.

9 *Subacute subdural haematoma.* More common in younger patients, with symptoms of persistent severe headache and vomiting, nausea, and drowsiness, culminating in a final serious deterioration in conscious level.

10 *Post-concussional symptoms* (headache, dizziness, depression, lack of concentration, and lethargy) are diagnosed by excluding other, more serious, complications, since all these symptoms are found in other conditions. Impairment of short-term memory and concentration and depression can make return to work difficult, and the opinion of a clinical psychologist on the need for a period of convalescence can help to prevent the patient being regarded as a malingerer.

Delayed symptoms (Box 12.1) following head injury are common after both serious injuries and relatively minor injuries. Indeed, the delayed complication may constitute a much more serious problem than the initial injury.

Box 12.1 Delayed complications of head injury

- Post-traumatic epilepsy
- Meningitis
- Aerocele
- Hydrocephalus
- Post-concussional syndrome
- Chronic subdural haematoma

Post traumatic epilepsy

Epilepsy may complicate both the relatively minor and the severe head injury. In the United States, approximately 500 000 patients are admitted to hospital with head injuries each year, and 30 000 (16%) have post-traumatic epileptic fits. An incidence of 5–7% has been reported in European studies. This development should not be taken to indicate that some new and sinister intracranial event has occurred. It does not, for instance, herald an intracranial haematoma, and does not alone, therefore, indicate urgent admission to a neurosurgical unit. Post-traumatic epileptic fits are described as **early**, when they occur within the first week following the injury, and **late**, when they occur after the first week.

In the case of **early epilepsy**, 30% occur within the first hour after injury, 30% in the subsequent 24 hours, and the remainder in the following week. Of early fits, 11% involve an episode of status epilepticus, and in children under the age of 5 years the incidence is as much as 20%. Early fits are more common after severe head injuries. A period of post-traumatic amnesia (PTA) of greater than 24 hours, depressed skull fractures, and intracranial haematomas are associated with an incidence of early epilepsy of 9–13%.

Late epilepsy occurs in approximately 5% of all head injuries (Box 12.2). The likelihood of the patient developing late (continuing) epilepsy depends on the nature of the injury, and can be roughly predicted. The incidence of late epilepsy is dependent on age, the severity of the injury, the occurrence of early epilepsy, and complications such as intracranial haematoma and depressed skull fracture.

The occurrence of early epilepsy is associated with an incidence of late epilepsy of 25%. If the head injury is complicated by extradural haematoma there is a 20% risk of late epilepsy, and the risk rises to 50% in the case of subdural and intracerebral haematoma. Depressed skull fracture is also associated with a high risk of epilepsy; but the risk is dependent on a number of other factors. Penetration of the dura, PTA of

---

Box 12.2   Factors associated with late epilepsy

- Early epilepsy
- Severe head injury
- Age < 5 years
- Intracranial haematoma
- Depressed skull fracture

greater than 24 hours, and early epilepsy all increase the risk. The combination of PTA greater than 24 hours, dural tear, and early epilepsy carries a risk of late fits of more than 60%. The severity of the head injury is defined by the duration of PTA. Post-traumatic amnesia of greater than 24 hours has a 25% risk of late fits.

Some 50% of late fits occur within one year of the injury; but a further 25% present after four years.

There is usually little difficulty in recognizing a classical **grand mal seizure**, and this is the commonest form of **early** fit. On the other hand, **partial seizures** may occur—taking the form of focal motor fits or absence attacks. In the latter, the patient becomes unresponsive for brief periods of time, and this may be misinterpreted as a progressive deterioration in conscious level if the abrupt onset is not recognized. Late post-traumatic fits often have a focal element, involving involuntary movement, sensory disturbance, or dysphasia, depending on the site of the injury.

No specific investigation is required when the patient is known to have had a fit following a head injury. The diagnosis is based on the doctor's observation of the incident or the account of witnesses. An electro-encephalogram (EEG) is of little value.

Management of post-traumatic fits with anticonvulsant drugs

The management of fits in the acute phase of the head injury is described on p. 52. Prophylactic anticonvulsant drugs have no influence on the development of late epilepsy. Anticonvulsants should be prescribed only if the patient has a fit, and must then be continued indefinitely if the patient wishes to reduce the likelihood of recurrent fits. The choice of drug is determined by the patient's age and sex. Phenytoin causes gum hyperplasia in children, and an alternative should be used. Sodium valproate should be avoided in women of child-bearing age, because of its teratogenic potential. The dose required in adults varies from one individual to another, and may have to be adjusted according to the success in controlling the fits and toxic side-effects. Doses in children are dependent on weight. Blood levels of phenytoin can be used to achieve therapeutic concentrations and to diagnose overdosage. They are unreliable for other drugs. Phenytoin, carbamazepine, and sodium valproate are the anticonvulsants of first choice. Phenobarbitone is an equally effective drug, but is more sedative than the others, and may cause hyperkinesia and behavioural disturbances in children. (See Box 12.3.)

Box 12.3 Anticonvulsant drugs

Phenytoin	200–300 mg/day
Carbamazepine	200 mg b.d., increasing to 800–1200 mg/day according to effect
Sodium valproate	600 mg/day in divided doses
Phenobarbitone	60 mg t.d.s.
Doses in children	according to weight

Meningitis

Meningitis is a complication of the penetrating head injury and the skull base injury. Penetrating injuries of the skull vault are usually clinically obvious, and if appropriately treated surgically are rarely complicated by infection. In the event of infection the commonest contaminating organism is *Staphylococcus aureus*.

Skull base fractures are less readily diagnosed Cerebrospinal fluid (CSF) rhinorrhoea or otorrhoea may be clinically obvious or occult, and may appear to have ceased when, in fact, the fistula persists but the CSF is being swallowed. Since the fracture involves the paranasal air sinuses or the mastoid air cells a variety of organisms may be responsible for infection. By far the most common form of meningitis complicating head injury is the **pneumococcal meningitis** complicating fractures of the anterior fossa and the middle third of the face, and fractures of the nasal bones. Prophylactic antibiotics are usually given for an arbitrary period after the injury or after the CSF leak has ceased. However, delayed meningitis may occur weeks, months, or years after such injuries, and the possibility of meningitis should be considered in patients who present with delayed symptoms after a known head injury.

Clinical features

The patient usually presents with a short history of progressive headache and *malaise*. Neck pain or back pain, photo-phobia, and vomiting are common symptoms. Drowsiness, confusion, and diplopia may follow. The characteristic physical signs are fever and neck stiffness, and these may be accompanied by reduced conscious level and focal neurological signs such as hemiparesis or cranial nerve palsies. Papilloedema may be found, particularly in the later stages of the disease.

Meningitis frequently progresses rapidly, and there is a high mortality rate, even when appropriate antibiotic therapy is started promptly. Early diagnosis is vital.

Diagnosis

Ideally, the diagnosis should be confirmed by lumbar puncture, and the nature and antibiotic sensitivity of the organism should be determined. A lumbar puncture should not be carried out if there is any suspicion of an intracranial mass, and, in these circumstances, a CT scan must be ordered first. This applies to patients with recent head injuries who have not fully recovered, and might therefore be harbouring an intracranial haematoma or cerebral contusion and to patients presenting with altered consciousness and/or papilloedema. If scanning facilities are not available, treatment must not be delayed, and antibiotic therapy must be started without a prior lumbar puncture. Before doing so blood should be taken for blood culture, and any nasal or aural discharge should be swabbed and sent for culture. A retrospective diagnosis may be possible if bacterial antigens can be detected by serology; but absence of bacterial antigens does not exclude the diagnosis of infection by a specific organism.

Treatment

As soon as specimens for bacteriological examination have been taken antibiotic therapy should be started. Until culture and sensitivity reports are available the treatment should cover all likely pathogens. When the patient is known to have had CSF rhinorrhoea or an anterior cranial fossa fracture **benzyl penicillin** must be given intravenously in high doses (2.4 g 4-hourly in adults; 180–300 mg/kg body weight in divided doses in children). If there has been CSF otorrhoea or a fracture of the petrous bone a variety of middle ear commensal organisms may cause meningitis, including Gram-negative and anaerobic species. Treatment should commence with **cefotaxime** (2 g 8-hourly; 100–150 mg/kg in divided doses in children) and **metronidazole** (500 mg 8-hourly; 7.5 mg/kg 8-hourly in children). It is wise to give all three antibiotics in combination until the causative organism and its sensitivity has been established. Antibiotic therapy must continue until the infection has been eradicated, and until any CSF fistula has been repaired. In the absence of a demonstrable CSF fistula antibiotic treatment should continue for at least 2 weeks; but if there is doubt about whether the infection has been eradicated the lumbar puncture should be repeated. If there is a persisting raised cell count in the CSF antibiotic treatment should continue.

Once the infection has been treated and the patient has made a full recovery the possibility of a CSF fistula must be investigated. There is a risk of recurrent meningitis if the fistula is not repaired.

> **Treatment of post-traumatic meningitis includes repair of the skull base fistula**

Aerocele

Anterior fossa skull base fractures may be complicated not only by the escape of cerebrospinal fluid (CSF), but also by air entering the anterior fossa. Since the brain may be adherent to the fracture site the air may form a 'balloon' in the frontal lobe, especially if air is blown in under force when the patient blows his nose. A large aerocele causes severe headache, usually of rapid onset. This may be accompanied by alteration of consciousness and focal deficits such as hemiparesis. Characteristically, this occurs in a patient who is recovering from the head injury, and the deterioration comes days or weeks later. In many instances a history linking the new symptoms to nose-blowing is not found, and the diagnosis is suggested by the nature of the original injury and the delayed deterioration.

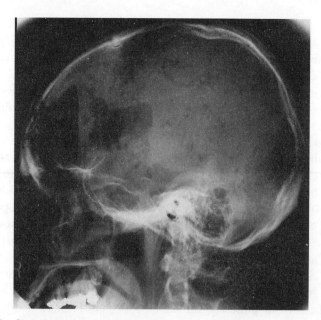

Fig. 12.1   Skull X-ray of an aerocele.

The diagnosis is easily made by plain brow-up skull X-rays, which show the collection of air in the anterior fossa (Fig. 12.1).

An aerocele will often resolve spontaneously; but this turn of events indicates that the patient has a significant fistula, which requires surgical repair to avert the possibility of meningitis. Antibiotic prophylaxis should be given.

Hydrocephalus

Hydrocephalus is a rare complication of head injury. It occurs more commonly after severe head injuries, and may be a cause of delayed deterioration or arrested recovery. Blood in the cerebrospinal fluid (CSF) may cause obstruction of CSF flow in the basal cisterns, or failure of CSF reabsorption in the sagittal sinus. This results in communicating hydrocephalus. The patient may make an unexpectedly slow recovery, or cease to recover. Alternatively, neurological deterioration may take place months or years after the head injury. The clinical features include headache, intellectual impairment, urinary incontinence, and gait disturbance. Papilloedema may occur, but is usually absent.

The diagnosis is made by CT scan. The finding of ventricular enlargement does not necessarily mean that the hydrocephalus is a result of trauma, however. Failure to recover as expected from a head injury may be due to pre-existing symptomless hydrocephalus, and treatment of the ventricular enlargement may not only be disappointing, but may also be complicated by acute subdural haematoma.

Chronic and subacute subdural haematoma

Chronic subdural haematoma is a condition that occurs most commonly in the elderly and in the alcoholic patient. In almost half these patients there is no previously recorded history of significant trauma. The pathophysiology of this condition appears to be related to venous haemorrhage from a bridging vein between the dura and the cortex. The possibility of this occurring is increased in those with cerebral atrophy and a greater interval between brain and dura. Instead of simply resolving, a membrane forms around the haematoma, and repeated haemorrhage from the highly vascular membrane leads to a gradual increase in the volume of the haematoma. The contents of the haematoma in the early stages are dark red, or black and tarry; but as time passes the fluid becomes dark brown, and then yellow, and more watery in consistency.

Where there is a known injury, there is often a period of weeks or even months before the patient presents with headache, intellectual deterioration, focal neurological signs such as hemiparesis or dysphasia, and deteriorating consciousness. Particularly in the elderly or alcoholic patient, this diagnosis is worth considering in the event of delayed deterioration after a head injury—even a relatively trivial one.

In younger patients venous haemorrhage of this sort tends to present more acutely in the form of the **subacute subdural haematoma**. The patient who has had a relatively minor injury fails to recover from the initial headache, and continues to complain of nausea, vomiting, and drowsiness. Focal neurological signs may be absent in the early stages; but the patient's condition deteriorates over days or even weeks, culminating in a final serious deterioration in the level of consciousness. The patient may have papilloedema. Drowsiness, focal neurological signs, persistent vomiting, and severe headache should make these patients readily distinguished from those with post-concussional symptoms.

Post-concussional syndrome

Post-concussional symptoms are very common after head injury cause anxiety among patients who have had minor concussional head injuries, and frequently lead to patients being reviewed in the A&E departments or in the general practitioner's surgery.

The most frequent complaints are of headache, 'dizziness', depression, lack of concentration, and lethargy. Each of these symptoms may be caused by other complications, and the diagnosis of 'post-concussional symptoms' is made by exclusion. Headache occurs in almost 70% of patients who are admitted to hospital after minor head injuries (post-traumatic amnesia > 24 hours), and roughly 30% of patients have headache that persists for more than 2 months. The headache is often related to exertion and fatigue, and is usually intermittent. Post-concussional headaches may be mild or severe. They are not accompanied by abnormal neurological signs. Dizziness is also a common complaint, and occurs in about 70% of cases. True vertigo is rare. Some impairment of short-term memory occurs in a similar number of patients.

A careful history must be taken, with particular reference to symptoms such as rhinorrhoea, drowsiness and intellectual impairment, neck pain, photophobia, and vomiting. The patient should be re-examined and the X-rays should be reviewed. It is neither practical nor desirable to order CT scans for the large number of patients who present with relatively minor symptoms following concussional injuries. The likelihood of symptoms being due to an intracranial haematoma is usually excluded by the time-scale. Extradural haematomas and acute subdural or intra-cerebral haematomas do not present after a delay of weeks, and almost invariably cause progressive neurological deterioration. Meningitis should also be readily recognizable from its characteristic symptoms and physical signs. In the elderly or alcoholic patient chronic subdural haematoma should be considered in the differential diagnosis, and there should be a greater readiness to order a CT scan in this group.

In the great majority of patients presenting with post-concussional symptoms, therefore, it is possible to make a clinical diagnosis and offer symptomatic treatment.

Treatment

The most important aspect of treatment is to explain the nature of the problem to the patient and to provide reassurance that the symptoms are not sinister, and will eventually resolve. Symptoms may persist for weeks or months. Depression may be responsive to antidepressant drugs.

Post-concussional symptoms may be associated with quite disabling intellectual impairment, although this may not be readily recognized on a cursory interview and examination. Impairment of short-term memory and concentration may make it very difficult for the patient to return to work; but the lack of obvious outward signs can lead to the patient being regarded as a malingerer. The opinion of a clinical psychologist can be invaluable in confirming that the patient is impaired, and should be allowed a period of convalescence.

Depression, anxiety, and lack of concentration may, on the other hand, be due more to the cause of the injury—to an impending court appearance or a violent spouse. Post-concussional symptoms, by definition, complicate a concussional injury, and are not the consequence of an injury that has not resulted in even a brief loss of consciousness.

Further reading

Friedman *et al.* (1945). Post traumatic vertigo and dizziness. *Journal of Neurosurgery*, **2**, 36–46.

Jennett, Bryan (1975). *Epilepsy after blunt head injury*. Heinemann Medical, Oxford.

Rimel, R. W. *et al.* (1981). Disability caused by minor head injury. *Neurosurgery*, **9**, 221–8.

Soroker *et al.* (1989) Practice of prophylactic anticonvulsant therapy in head injury. *Brain Injury*, **3**, 137–40.

13 Transporting the head-injured patient

Chapter contents

Key points in transporting head-injured patients

1   Indications for urgent transfer to a neurosurgical centre are: persisting altered consciousness after resuscitation; deteriorating conscious level; altered consciousness accompanied by skull fracture; head-injured patient requiring ventilation; compound depressed skull fracture. An early epileptic fit is not, in itself, an indication for transfer.
2   The patient should be fully resuscitated and in a stable cardiorespiratory state before transfer.
3   The decision to transfer should be made by a senior doctor. The receiving doctor will require details of the type of injury, conscious level and any change in conscious level, pupil size and reaction, cardiorespiratory status, and other injuries.
4   Consider whether the patient should be ventilated prior to transfer; consider whether a diuretic should be given.
5   Any patient with a Glasgow Coma Score of 8 or less should be ventilated prior to transfer.
6   The unconscious patient should be accompanied by an experienced doctor, preferably an anaesthetist.
7   Pulse, blood pressure, ECG, oxygen saturation and end-tidal carbon dioxide monitoring should be used in transfer.

The head-injured patient may require referral to a neurosurgical unit or intensive care unit for further investigation and treatment. Transportation of the critically ill patient involves potential risks to both the patient and the transfer team. It is important to have a clear understanding of the indications for referral and the ideal conditions required for a safe transfer.

Secondary referral of head-injured patients

Secondary referral is indicated either when the patient requires specialist neurosurgical attention or when the head-injured patient has other injuries requiring specialist attention not available in the base hospital. (See Box 13.1.)

Referral to a neurosurgical centre may be indicated because the patient currently has an injury requiring neurosurgical supervision and specialist neurosurgical nursing, or because complications of the head injury are anticipated. In the first group are patients with severe primary brain injuries, patients with deteriorating consciousness following head injury, and patients with skull or scalp injuries requiring operative treatment. It is important to remember that a common cause of deterioration in con-

Box 13.1   Indications for urgent transfer to a neurosurgical centre

After resuscitation

- Persistent coma
- Deteriorating conscious level
- Focal neurological signs

Fractured skull with:

- Any alteration in conscious level
- Focal neurological signs

Compound depressed skull fracture
Head injury requiring ventilation

scious level after head injury are systemic factors—principally respiratory impairment and hypotension.

The second group of patients are those who may not have suffered a severe primary injury but in whom secondary brain injury is anticipated—most commonly as a result of intracranial haematoma. Thus, the patient who has a skull fracture and persisting altered consciousness after resuscitation is known to face a 25% risk of some form of intracranial haematoma and requires a computerized tomography (CT) scan and, possibly, the opinion of a neurosurgeon. This may involve the transfer of the patient to a distant hospital. When air ambulance transfer is required, a further factor influencing the timing of transfer may be available daylight and the weather conditions.

Secondary referral may also be necessary for the management of other injuries when suitable facilities are not available at the base hospital. Patients with severe facial injuries, chest injuries, and those with multiple injuries may require assisted ventilation. Once the patient is ventilated no further clinical monitoring of the neurological condition is possible. In these circumstances, the patient must have a CT scan and, if there is evidence of significant intracranial trauma, intracranial pressure monitoring will be required in order to recognize and treat increasing intracranial mass in the form of progressive haematoma or brain swelling.

An early epileptic fit is not in itself a reason for immediate referral since this is not, in isolation, an indication that the patient is developing an intracranial haematoma.

Before the transfer is accepted there must be adequate communication at a senior level. The decision to transfer should be made jointly by the referring doctor and the receiving doctor. The receiving unit will need information about the patients current neurological condition and any change in conscious level that has taken place since the injury (Box 13.2). Conscious level must be described in the terms of the Glasgow Coma Scale. The referring doctor should be able to describe the pupils size and reaction to light and the patient's current pulse rate and blood pressure. The receiving unit will wish to establish that resuscitation has been completed and that the patient has had X-rays of the chest and cervical spine. In order to allow the receiving hospital to alert the relevant specialties, the nature and extent of other injuries should be described.

In consultation with the neurosurgeon, it must be decided whether the patient should be ventilated prior to transfer and whether a diuretic agent (20% **mannitol** or **frusemide**) should be given.

The transfer

Transport from the scene of the accident

The commonest causes of secondary brain injury are hypoxia and hypotension. At the scene of the accident the airway must be cleared and secured for the journey. A high concentration of oxygen should be administered by face mask. External bleeding should be controlled by pressure and the cervical spine must be immobilized.

Care must be taken not to cause further intracranial hypertension by applying tight collars or tapes round the neck. The patient should not be tilted head-down in the course of the journey. Acceleration forces have been reported to cause reduction of cardiac output and might, theoretically, have an adverse effect on cerebral perfusion. A smooth journey at a steady speed is preferable to a very fast journey with periods of acceleration and deceleration.

Helicopter transport (air ambulance) is being used increasingly in some countries in place of road ambulances. There are a number of advantages in using a helicopter. Acceleration can be controlled more smoothly and is only required at the beginning of the flight. A much less bumpy ride is possible. If the patient is transported feet-first, the effects of acceleration are counteracted by the nose-down tilt of the helicopter and the head-up tilt of the patient. Wherever possible, the patient with a serious head injury should be taken directly to a trauma centre equipped with all the trauma specialties rather than to the nearest hospital.

Secondary transfer from the admitting hospital

During secondary transfer of head-injured patients the level of care given should be no less than that given before and after transfer. For this to be

Box 13.2   Information required by the receiving unit

- Type and time of injury
- Conscious level after injury
- Change in conscious level
- Pupil size and reaction
- Focal neurological signs
- Cardiorespiratory status: blood pressure pulse, respiratory rate, arterial blood gases
- Other injuries
- Management and response to date

accomplished a great deal of planning and preparation must take place both in terms of staff training, organization, and the funding and purchase of equipment. Hospitals that are involved in transfers of head-injured patients should have clear guidelines for arrangements for initiating and carrying out transfers.

The transfer itself can be a hazardous experience for both the patient and accompanying personnel and it is essential that those who are accompanying patients are properly trained and experienced in the environments that they will encounter. Physiological risks arise not only from the patients condition but also from the effects of movement (tipping, vibration, acceleration/deceleration forces), changes in barometric pressure and changes in temperature.

Environments such as the back of a speeding ambulance or the dark, noisy belly of a helicopter are not ones in which adequate resuscitation can be achieved. It is vital that the patient's condition should have been stabilized and resuscitation completed prior to the commencement of transfer.

There will always be situations where it may be prudent to expedite a transfer but only if there are clear benefits from the treatment offered by the receiving unit.

A number of studies have shown a high incidence of secondary brain insults due to hypoxia and hypotension during secondary transfer of severely head-injured patients. Similar observations have been made of inter-hospital transfer (e.g. for CT scan). Gentleman and Jennett (1981) reported that 45% of unconscious patients transferred to a neurosurgical unit were inadequately resuscitated before or during transfer. Complications during transfer have been shown to occur more commonly when the patient is escorted by a junior and inexperienced doctor.

> **The patient's condition must be stabilized and resuscitation completed before transfer**

The decision that a patient is ready for transfer requires experience and should follow a period of observation in the resuscitation room. This can legitimately delay transfer. It cannot be overstressed that transfer must not start until the patient's condition is stable.

Staff

Those accompanying head-injured patients must be trained. Ideally, there should be at least one doctor and one nurse. Current recommendations are that the doctor should have received training in intensive care and transport medicine. They are fully responsible for the care of the patient during transfer and so must be able to deal with any problem that might arise. They must not leave the hospital until they are fully conversant with the history, treatment, and current status and are certain that resuscitation has been completed.

Preparation for transfer

The criteria for endotracheal intubation and ventilation are shown in Box 13.3. If the patient has not already been intubated, serious consideration should be given to doing so prior to transfer. The need for intubation during a transfer indicates inadequate assessment and preparation prior to leaving the base hospital and is substandard practice.

As well as familiarizing themselves with the patient, the transfer team should have meticulously checked and be familiar with all the equipment and drugs they are taking with them. They should ensure that all monitoring equipment is functioning, with adequate back-up battery supplies. Intravenous lines, the urinary catheter, and the endotracheal tube must be secured by tapes. They should be familiar with the operation of monitoring and resuscitation equipment supplied in the vehicle. They should be familiar with the contents of the resuscitation bags and the workings and limitations of portable ventilators and defibrillators.

The transfer team should have a means of communication such as a portable phone and, for their own comfort, money and warm clothing.

Box 13.3   Indications for intubation and ventilation after head injury

Immediate

- Coma (Glasgow Coma Score < 8)
- Loss of protective laryngeal reflexes
- Respiratory inadequacy (by arterial blood gases)
  - Hypoxaemia (PaO_2 < 9 kPa on air; < 13 kPa on oxygen)
  - Hypercarbia ($PaCO_2$ > 6 kPa)
- Spontaneous hyperventilation causing $PaCO_2$ < 3.5 kPa
- Irregular respiration

Before start of transfer

- Significant deterioration in conscious level
- Bilateral fractured mandible/severe facial injury
- Epileptic fits

All intubated patients must receive adequate sedation and be ventilated with muscle relaxation
Aim for PaO_2 > 13 kPa; $PaCO_2$ 4.0–4.5 kPa

Prior to leaving the referring unit, go through the equipment checklist (Box 13.4) and review the patient's condition. Inform the receiving unit of the expected time of arrival.

Box 13.4   Essential transfer equipment check list

- Airways and endotracheal tubes
- Facemasks and self-inflating AMBU bag
- Back-up oxygen supply
- Portable suction machine
- Laryngoscopes, cannulae, and intravenous fluids
- Portable ventilator
- ECG, blood pressure, pulse oximeter, end-tidal CO_2 monitors
- Supply of drugs (sedatives, relaxants, emergency resuscitation drugs)
- Battery-operated syringe pumps
- Warming blankets
- Case notes, recordings, X-rays
- Warm clothing, money, portable phone

Transfer of the deteriorating head-injured patient

If the patient's conscious level had deteriorated after admission to hospital despite adequate resuscitation, there must be suspicion of a developing intracranial haematoma. It is essential to make every effort to control intracranial pressure (ICP) until definitive surgical measures can be taken. Irreparable secondary damage may occur in the hours required to arrange and undertake transfer to a neurosurgical centre. Within this group of patients are those who might expect a good quality of recovery if they can be brought to operative neurosurgical treatment sufficiently early.

Intracranial pressure is controlled by two measures. First, intubation and positive pressure ventilation ensure that the $PaCO_2$ is controlled and that hypoxia is avoided. This, in turn, prevents cerebral hyperaemia and consequent intracranial hypertension. It is essential, if this is to be done, that the patient is paralysed and sedated throughout the journey. Coughing and making respiratory efforts against the ventilator exacerbate raised ICP. Second, ICP can be lowered by the administration of diuretic agents. The one most commonly used is **mannitol**. This should be given as a bolus in the form of 20% **mannitol**. The dose is 0.5 g/kg body weight (i.e. approximately 200 ml of 20% **mannitol** in an average adult). **Frusemide** is a suitable alternative.

These measures will 'buy' a period of grace of 2 hours at most, and no time must be lost in arranging transfer while these temporary stabilizing measures are being taken. If the patient is not already catheterized a urinary catheter should be passed. Neurological monitoring after paralysis and sedation is, of course, largely impossible. The only evidence of deterioration as a result of a rise in ICP might be the development of pupil asymmetry. In that event, a further bolus of **mannitol** should be given. (See Box 13.5.)

Box 13.5   Actions to take when transferring the deteriorating head-injured patient

- Intubate and ventilate
- Ensure sedation and complete paralysis
- Intravenous **mannitol** 20% : 0.5 mg/kg body weight

OR

- Intravenous **frusemide**
- Urinary catheter
- Rapid transfer

Further reading

Bristow, J. and Toff, N. J. (1992). A report: Recommended standards for UK fixed wing medical air transport systems and for patient management during transfer by fixed wing aircraft. *Journal of the Royal Society of Medicine*, **85**, 767–71.

Gentleman, D. (1990). Audit of transfer of unconscious patients to a Neurosurgical Unit. *Lancet*, **335**, 330–4.

Gentleman, D. and Jennett, B. (1981). Hazards of inter-hospital transfer of comatose head injured patients. *Lancet*, **2**, 853–5.

Gentleman, D., Drearden, M., Midgely, S., and Maclean, D. (1993). Guidelines for the resuscitation and transfer of patients with serious head injury. *British Medical Journal*, **307**, 547–52.

Intensive Care Society (November, 1997). *Guidelines for the transport of the critically ill adult*. Intensive Care Society, London.

Jeffries, N. and Bristow, A. (1991). Long distance inter-hospital transfers (helicopter transport). *British Journal of Intensive Care*, **1**, 197–203.

The Neuroanaesthesia Society of Great Britain and Ireland (1996). *Recommendations for the transfer of patients with acute head injuries to neurosurgical units*. The Association of Anaesthetists of Great Britain and Ireland, London.

Wright, I. H. *et al.* (1988). Provision of facilities for secondary transport of severely ill patients in the United Kingdom. *British Medical Journal*, **296**, 543–5.

Index